Living Hell to Living Well

John Awen

GREEN MAGIC

Green Magic
53 Brooks Road
Street
Somerset
BA16 0PP
England

www.greenmagicpublishing.com

Designed and typeset by
K.DESIGN, Winscombe, Somerset

ISBN 9781916014091

GREEN MAGIC

Contents

Foreword

'What do you want to be when you grow up?' An impossible question for most kids, but not me. From a very young age, I was certain that I was going to be a doctor and spend my working life making people better. Fast forward a couple of decades and a million exams, and there I was, a qualified medical professional all set to live my dream.

But here's the thing. I quickly realised that a lot of the time I wasn't making people better. Often I was, with pain relief, or antibiotics for example, but mostly my job involved slowing disease down – people still got sicker, just more slowly, something I was (and still am) so grateful to be able to do for them with modern medicine, but twenty years of training taught me that chronic diseases like heart disease, diabetes, arthritis and many more don't 'get better', they only ever get worse.

I had more questions than answers, so I went back to the medical literature, and to University for a nutrition degree, and it turns out that the evidence I was searching for was already there, hidden in plain sight. Heart disease is potentially reversible. There are no guarantees, but potentially reversible nonetheless, and our diets are a major factor in determining whether our arteries get more or less clogged up as time passes. And the diet with the best evidence in terms of reversing heart disease is the one that John writes about in this book, and the one that I personally follow and advise my patients to adopt; a whole food, plant-based diet.

I cannot recommend this book highly enough; even if you have no interest in a plant-based diet, John's tale of triumph over adversity is truly remarkable and as unique as he is, and is a gripping, white-knuckle roller-coaster ride with twists and turns that I could never have imagined! I read it in one sitting because I simply could not put it down. But I also entirely agree with his dietary choices, and I've tried some of his recipes – they are simple and delicious, as all food should be!

One aspect of this book, however, is not unique. Increasing numbers of people are realising the power of a plant-based diet to heal heart disease and many other conditions, and are getting results like John has. If you haven't already, please consider trying it for yourself – you have nothing to lose, and who knows just what you might gain?

Dr Sue Kenneally MBBS MRCGP MSc ANutr

GP, nutritionist, lifestyle physician

Introduction

Within the pages of this book, I am going to take you on an incredible journey, one which will resonate fully within you, amaze and leave you dumbstruck in parts. I will plant seeds within you, and make you question all that you thought you knew. In a nutshell; I will turn your world and your beliefs upside down.

We live many lives within this one, some good and some not so good, although what truly matters in all of this is how we rise and meet the challenges that this life will invariably throw at us.

From an early age, I always questioned life and searched for the answers. I have hit the self-destruct button many times, as I am sure many people have done. I openly admit that my self-destruction has been to the extreme and has seen me plunged into some of the darkest depths imaginable. Yet having climbed out of the dark pit of despair and totally turned my life around, I now share openly and candidly, and in doing so I hope that I can reach, touch and inspire others who may be struggling and finding life tough.

Nobody ever said this life would be easy. It's tough, and not just for us, but for all beings. It is from this understanding, coupled with an intrinsic knowledge of the complexities faced by all species, that I have managed personally to reach and follow a place within myself where heartfelt compassion and empathy are key and my guiding forces within this life.

With a brief journey into my formative and early years I will tell the main points in my life, describe the darkness involved with a long-term heroin addiction and the shocking truths of that journey. I will tell my tale of how I became clean, the knock-on health effects from that time and how I managed to totally turn my life around from that point.

From living on a smallholding, feeding, caring for and helping animals give birth, to then eventually leading the same animals onto the kill room floor of a slaughterhouse and watching what happens. Between my indoctrinated mindset and my breaking heart at what I was doing, it was this and other experiences that led me to becoming Vegan and abstaining, as much as is humanly possible, from allowing animal cruelty in my name.

Travel with me as I explain what it is like to be told I shouldn't be waking up each morning as my heart was so severely damaged, feel the despair as I did.

From being prescribed life-saving medication for all of the heart ailments to striving to bring about the much needed changes within my own health by adopting a WFPB (whole foods plant-based) diet and eventually eating my way to being free of heart disease and medication free.

Now, as well as being a multiple published author, I am a public speaker and a qualified Vegan/plant-based nutritionist and I am living proof that no matter what we encounter upon this journey of life, we can ultimately change, and people do all the time.

It is often within our darkest and most oppressive times that great strength and clarity are found and received. From that point, the onus falls upon us to think, act and start becoming the best version of ourselves that we can be.

Forget all that you thought you knew about healthy eating and all that gives us strong, healthy teeth and bones.

I will introduce you to a way of living that anatomically we are totally equipped for. I will myth-bust and scientifically, medically and environmentally slay the myths which have built up around Veganism and a plant-based way of life.

With fact based links that you can reference and cross check, medical evidence from some of the world's most prolific plant-based doctors, scientifically proven docu-mentaries that are readily and easily accessible online for you to watch, plus my own journey which saw me diagnosed with advanced heart failure in mid-2015, where I was given no time to live at all, a journey which saw me taking copious amounts of prescribed medication, to now being totally medication free and with several of my heart conditions showing signs of reversal and others no further deterioration.

Hold on tight as you embark on this journey which will be rounded off with several recipes from me, as I am also a fully qualified Vegan nutritionist.

Within the upcoming pages, I will give you a life story, although not a mundane one. I will not bore you with trivial parts which have no relevance, plus with 51 years of life behind me, you don't want to hear about it all, and in all honesty, I don't have 51 years to write every aspect of my life. So what I will do is give you precise, key facts and the main bullet point moments and times of my life that have been pivotal in bringing me to who and what I am now.

I sincerely hope that you enjoy the words within this book and that it will give you an insight into my life and show to you that, no matter how tough life gets, change is always possible, we just have to want it and be prepared to work extremely hard to achieve it.

Openly and candidly sharing my journey from darkness into light, I tell my own personal tale with hard hitting truths and facts. Even when I had emerged from heroin addiction, the health implications were huge and, ultimately, saw me being told that I had no time to live, as my heart was so severely damaged.

From this realisation I began a slow process of looking for ways to maybe heal my own heart and reverse the heart disease I was diagnosed with.

A gradual process which culminated in me reversing several of the heart conditions I had, also allowed me to gradually wean myself off of the various life-saving medications I was prescribed and taking twice a day.

With various websites and findings from several of the world's most prolific plant-based doctors, the facts are all there for everyone to see.

If you would like to contact me, then feel free to connect via my website:

www.johnawen.com

Thank you and enjoy the journey within
the forthcoming pages.

Acknowledgements

Life is a very rich and wondrous gift, a tapestry that we create along the way, some plucks in the thread and some beautiful and very rich colourations as well. For no matter what may befall us upon this journey, what ultimately matters is how we rise up to face the challenges, wade through them, then learn and evolve and become the very best version of ourselves that we can.

We often choose to stand alone on this journey, we all have our own thoughts and we live our own lives, but it is those around us though that we have to thank for their constant and invaluable support, no matter whether times are good, or not so.

True friends can never be lost, they are there for us, always willing to listen and offer advice, it is these beautiful souls that we all need in our lives, much credit and respect to them all, here are a few I would like to give a shout out to:

Pete Gotto, my publisher at Green Magic Publishing, for not only has he published all five of my books, he is also a great friend and often proves to be a font of knowledge.

SR Photography who captured brilliantly the back cover, 'One Dog and His Man,' and also some of the images used within this book.

Dr Sue Kennealy, for agreeing to write the foreword for this book. She has been an inspiration and a great source of comfort and insight to many in her vocation as a GP and a plant-based doctor.

Jennifer Justice, such an amazing friend and human being and her tireless work in raising awareness of the cruelty committed upon dolphins, whales and other aquatic life which is inspirational.

Jay, Luke and their beautiful son Idan, a family of incredibly special souls who I am proud to call my friends, who have been there for me on several occasions. They own and run the company 'Viva La Vegan,' which creates ethical, sustainable and inspirational animal activist apparel and other merchandise. I am honoured to be their ambassador and I can always be seen wearing their innovative range of clothing.

Shirley and Derrick Tregonning, a lovely husband and wife team who I am proud to know and call friends. Together they set up two ethical Vegan businesses, one of which is called 'There's No Catch,' which serves delicious plant-based and Vegan street food and they also have 'There's No Whey,' which serves the very best dairy free ice-cream. I am immensely proud to also be the ambassador for both of these cruelty free and sustainable companies.

Caroline and Chelsea, a mother and daughter who created Herbipaws, a game changing company which sells cruelty free and plant-based dog treats and once again, I am so proud to be an ambassador for them.

A massive thank you to my friend Philip Wollen for taking the time out of his busy schedule to write the very heart warming endorsement for this book.

Philip is one of the most inspirational and influential people I know and I am proud to know him and be standing with him on the right side of history.

Thank you to Jane Tredgett, who set up Humane Being company and then the campaign Scrap Factory Farming, which will undoubtedly set a precedent as it seeks to help end all that is wrong in this world.

I am very honoured to know Jane and am very proud to be an Ambassador for both Humane being and the Scrap Factory Farming campaign.

My very precious and most beautiful companion dog Pagan. In 2011 I went to view a different dog to rescue. Pagan, or Payton as he was then, chose me and since then, he has saved my life many times. He has always been there with me, through heartache and the absolute best of times. The day he chose me was, on reflection, like winning the jackpot. Pagan has shown and taught me some of the most powerful lessons I have and will ever learn in this lifetime, the greatest of those was to live in the moment and live each day as if it is your last and take nobody or anything for granted.

To all the countless people who have believed in me, supported me from afar and inspired me along my journey of life, thank you all so much.

The many people who have laughed at me, judged me and criticised me in what I do, I thank you also as you made me try even harder and helped me evolve into the best version of myself.

Thank you and much love to every one of you.

The Formative Years

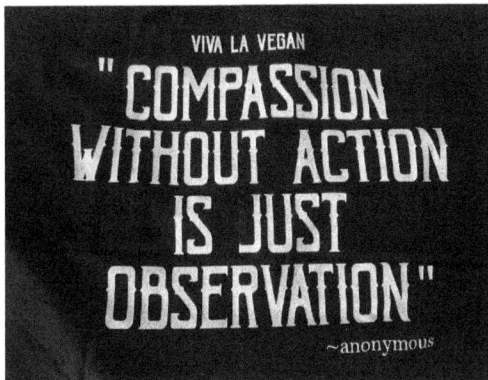

VIVA LA VEGAN

" COMPASSION WITHOUT ACTION IS JUST OBSERVATION "

~anonymous

I was born in the early hours, 5:20am of a Tuesday morning in 1969 in Colchester, Essex. Delivered by C – section as there were complications, the umbilical cord that attached me to my mum was wrapped around my neck and with further investigation it was discovered I had a serious water infection and also had underdeveloped lungs.

Nowadays these are not deemed as life threatening as they were back then. Due to this, I was placed in an incubator and put onto the critical list. I was being fed through a tube, receiving various medications through tubes and was being aided with my breathing. During this time I was devoid of any physical contact as I was seriously vulnerable and not expected to make it, so much so that both my parents were told several times to go and say goodbye to me.

I remained in that incubator for between 8–9 weeks. Needless to say, I pulled through and this survival must have been ingrained within me from those starting moments as doggedness, tenacity and being one of life's survivors has been a massive part of my life. To this day, I am still rising up, more often than not, against the odds.

Family life was good whilst growing up and was what I would class as 'normal,' I was the younger of two children and our family was not rich, not by any means. We lived in a council house but there was always food to eat, clean clothes to wear and presents for birthdays and Christmas, so I have no complaints there at all.

Both my parents are passed away now and I have not had any contact with my sister for over twenty years. This suits us both fine as we are polar opposites and our lives took massively different turns as is often the case within families, especially siblings.

From an early age, I knew I was different. I could never switch my mind off and I was always plaguing my parents, teachers, anybody really with questions, such was the extent of my ever enquiring and inquisitive mindset.

This must have driven my parents, my mum especially, to despair as, at aged 7 years old, I was forced to attend Sunday school which was at the village church where I lived in Sible Hedingham, Essex.

I actually enjoyed being read stories from the Bible each Sunday as myself and other young children sat cross legged on the floor with our relevant teachers for the lesson.

This excitement soon wore off as after each scripture reading I had a multitude of questions and must have driven the teachers there crazy as my incessant questioning never ceased, so much so that after a few weeks I became the invisible child and was being ignored. Hindsight shows me that these teachers and adults who were in charge didn't have the answers I was seeking, so it was easier to ignore me, sad really but it was what it was, and I hold no blame at all.

These experiences and situations are all relevant and have played a huge part in my life and who I am today. So, if you are pondering as to why I am writing this, it will all become clear and apparent the further into my life we venture as to why I became who I became, and also as to why I have slumped into some dark places.

After what seemed an eternity at that tender age and was probably around one year or maybe just over, I told my mum that I was allowed to take the family dog to church with me each Sunday. Whether she believed me or not was never discussed, but each Sunday I would take our family dog, a Jack Russell Terrier named Judy, out of the house at the relevant Sunday school times.

I headed off into the woods instead and then returned home for dinner, again at the time I would have returned if I had been attending the church.

Hindsight shows me now that it was during these times that nature became my church and as well as climbing trees, making small dens for Judy and myself to sit in, I would talk out loud. These were inner frustrations, questions and longings to know the depth of life and the Universe and it is apparent now that I was asking a higher power, god/goddess/deity for answers. This helped me immensely, as I sought peace and solitude away from others; again, this has played a huge part in making me who and what I am now, and has served me well.

Hopes and Dreams

Growing up was good, special memories indeed. Living where we did ensured that there was always something to do; woods, rivers, ponds, old bomb shelters and other areas where children like to play and spend time in.

School was ok, I excelled at certain lessons, although these were subjects which I enjoyed and could actually see the sense in why I was being taught them. Whereas topics that didn't appeal to me I just didn't bother with, this trait which was so prevalent within me, even at the age of seven years, has stayed within me and still forms a massive part of who and what I am today.

There was one teacher who I would like to thank, Miss West was her name. She instilled within me my absolute passion for the English language at the tender age of seven years old.

A very spindly lady, who is long since dead, as she was old or certainly appeared it back in the mid-seventies. Then again, at such a young age, everybody appears old. She wore glasses that were always balanced precariously on the tip of her nose and a bun in her hair, appearing almost witch-like.

Without Miss West making learning fun and being so stoic in her teaching of the English language, there is no doubt in my mind whatsoever that I would not have become a published author. I have such a passion within me for writing and orating, so a massive thank you to her for being a guiding light in my younger years and such a huge influence on me.

I remember clearly one very dark, grey and wet Friday afternoon in her class as we played 'cricket with a difference' and I really looked forward to this game. Someone from the class would stand at the blackboard, as we had in those days, they would be in bat and members of the class would take it in turns to effectively bowl to them, the bowling was done with words. The child in bat would then have to use chalk to spell the words bowled at them on the blackboard. If they spelled correctly, another word from a different member of the class would be bowled at them. If spelt wrongly, that child who was in bat was then classed as out and another class member would step up to take the batting position.

It was during this that, when I was in bat, I was asked to spell 'writer,' which I did and ended by saying, "one day I will be a writer and have books published." This resonates deeply within me as this was obviously an insight into what was to come. Since the age of three years old I had always wanted to become a soldier and join the army. So on that Friday afternoon, for me to say that, it totally threw me as writing, even though I really enjoyed it, had never been on my radar at all and this was the only time I ever deviated from my longing to join the army.

School carried on as it does. I, as many of us do, endured it and enjoyed parts of it, although I longed to be free from the subservience and rulings. Again, this is another powerful trait which has stuck within me and only gotten stronger with age and maturity.

I finally left schooling in May 1985 and the qualifications I gained were in English language, maths, history and woodwork. No surprise there really as these were the only lessons I attended and applied myself to.

Shattered Dreams

Having dreamed of an army career since I was three years old, I visited the army careers office in Colchester, Essex and attended a few meetings with them there in late 1986 and early 1987. I later passed a basic test and was accepted into the REME (Royal Electrical and Mechanical Engineers) and my date for joining up and starting my basic training was set for February 1988. Everything that I had dreamed of was finally in place. It was with hidden pride, and trepidation, that I was so looking forward to becoming a soldier, as this was what I wanted to do and had longed for all my life.

On October 23, 1987 I was out early in the morning on my motorbike, I had a Suzuki 125cc and I was off to Sudbury in Suffolk to do some shopping for my mum.

It was a dry day and I was enjoying the early morning ride out. As I was leaving the village where I lived, I approached a junction on the left as a bright yellow mini metro started pulling out, I moved to the centre of the road to avoid the car, but it just pulled out and I went straight into the side. All I remember after that is the actual impact and deafening noise.

The next thing I remember is being in hospital. I had been taken there by ambulance and due to the severity of my injuries, a shattered left ankle; I had been given heavy pain relief whilst in the ambulance which is why I remember none of the journey or arrival at the hospital.

It transpired that they were seriously considering amputating my foot, it was so badly broken. Luckily, after reviews from several different surgeons, the decision was made to plate my ankle and, after a long surgical procedure, my left ankle received a plate, ten screws and various bits of wire in it.

I remained in Colchester General Hospital for nine days following the accident. Once I left, little did I know how much my life had changed and would propel me onto the longest, and often darkest, periods of my life.

On arriving home, my journey to recovery was extremely slow and incredibly painful. I had a three-quarter length plaster cast on my left leg and had been given a pair of old wooden under the arm crutches to manoeuvre around on; the total frustration from all of this was harrowing to say the least.

After a couple of months, having notified the army of my accident, I received notification from them to say that, due to the severity of my injuries, I would not be accepted into the army as the injuries were so great that that basic training would not be allowed, so all I had dreamed of was over.

Clumps of my hair started to fall out due to alopecia, such was from the shock my body and mind had received, I went off my food, which for me had never happened before.

As the weeks and months passed by, I can honestly say that these were tough times, as I had had my dreams and goals removed. I had absolutely no idea as to what to do next and I was not equipped to figure out my next move and which direction to take.

What apparently should have been around four to six months of using crutches, through my own stupidity and stubbornness, turned into just over a year as I kept trying to walk unaided. This was out of total frustration more than anything. I also had two minor surgeries during this time, again on my ankle to tighten up the screws as I had, apparently, loosened them due to attempting to walk unaided; totally my own fault.

By the end of 1988 I was finally free of the crutches but lacked motivation for pretty much everything. I was introduced to cannabis around this time and I have to admit, this really helped at the time as it assisted me in switching off my highly active and ever enquiring mind.

The days and months passed by in a haze of cannabis smoking, plus, as time passed, I found myself not only taking cannabis, but also using large amounts of speed and dabbling with LSD.

It was during mid 1989 that I sank to an exceptionally low point; I had obtained a large amount of morphine tablets and various tranquilisers and decided I had had enough, so I took the whole lot.

My mum (bless her heart and R.I.P.) had found me and could not wake me up, so she had called an ambulance. I was taken, once again, to Colchester General Hospital where I was stomach-pumped, which they did in those days. Because of this, and due to the procedures back then, as it was not an accidental overdose, I was sectioned for a deliberate overdose. The section was for 72 hours and I spent those three days in Severalls Hospital in Colchester, a secure hospital for patients with severe mental health problems, it has now long since closed.

As if I didn't feel bad enough beforehand, obviously as I had tried to take my own life, now I found myself in a secure unit with people who had major issues and problems. To say this was an incredibly low point in my life would be a huge understatement.

Upon release from this secure unit, I felt even more lost than I had before. Feelings of total frustration, confusion, bitterness and many other emotions and feelings consumed me totally at every waking moment, also many sleepless nights saw me contemplating the meaning of life and considering what a release death would be.

Eventually I started drifting from one job to another, builder's labourer, painter and decorator, etc. Whatever I did I simply could not apply myself. Effectively I was just existing and I continued to use large amounts of so-called recreational drugs which, on hindsight, only made matters worse. Although, at the time I thought they were helping me and allowing my mind to be at peace. How wrong I was.

The months and years became a blur fuelled by smoking cannabis continually and, I suppose, looking and hoping for a way out as, I remember thinking then, there must be more to life, as I was gripped in an uneventful stasis of mere existence and inner loathing.

Addiction and Alleged Offences

Addicts are not an elitist group. I am not going to glorify addiction, for it is a very dark place indeed, and nobody is exempt from the grips of it.

We live in a world where cigarette smoking, the drinking of alcohol and other vices are, for the mainstream, accepted. Frowned upon by the few, yet partaken of by the majority. Heroin is different, a small percentage fall into its vice-like clutches and the majority see them and view them with horror, disdain and often total contempt.

Nobody sets out to become an addict. Yet, once there, it is a mere existence; a constant battle. The statistics are frightening, so I will show you the stats and then allow you an insight into the absolute hell on earth that I experienced for eleven years before finally breaking free from the restraints that heroin held me in.

Long term heroin addiction is seen as the period of between two to five years. Once you hit this time scale, only around 3% of users actually break free and stay free for the rest of their lives. Whereas the other 97% die, either as a direct result of their addiction, or remain addicts for life and die from other causes. Either way, these are heart breaking facts and more needs to be done to stem these terrible numbers and help those who have drastically lost their way in life.

Nobody is exempt from addiction, regardless of which guise it may take. Maybe a job loss, a divorce; there are a multitude of reasons that can turn a person's life upside down to such a degree that they feel the need to hide themselves away from society behind a smokescreen of addiction that shields them from the real world and from themselves. So, we all need to view the bigger picture in all of this; be thankful it is not you and learn not to judge others.

In mid-1997 I was feeling totally lost. I had no anchors in my life, was unable to find a release for my ever questioning and insatiably inquisitive mind and had recently been acquitted in Chelmsford Crown Court of a conspiracy to purchase and supply £10,000 worth of amphetamine sulphate. This charge had been weighing heavily on my mind for over two years as, even though I was out on bail, albeit with strict conditions, had I been found guilty I would have received a prison sentence, which at that time would have been between five and eight years.

This had all stemmed from a police raid at a premise where

I had been present and a kilo of amphetamine sulphate had been discovered and I had been arrested for this. The fact is that the property I was in at the time, where the narcotics were found, was not even mine. So, to cut a long story short, after around two years of constant police harassment at every opportunity they could find, I was acquitted on all counts and it was actually revealed in Crown Court that Essex Police had been acting illegally and unscrupulously, which sadly was often the case back then.

Another example of police bias towards me at this time was when I was arrested for a dangerous driving offence, for which I was not guilty. Yet, on the court date, out of nowhere three Police officers were prepared to testify in court and swear they had all seen me driving a car that matched one of the cars I owned. The long and short of this is that I had no choice but to plead guilty.

I became the first person in Essex, in early 1995 to be disqualified under what was then a new law. This meant that anybody who was convicted of either dangerous driving, or drink driving, would be banned from driving for a fixed period, mine was three years. To start driving again after this, I would need to retake the driving test.

Introduction to Heroin

My dark and self-destructive journey into, and with, heroin began in mid-1997. As I previously mentioned; there had been many various reasons why I had become so lost and basically all these various parts had built up inside of me and I had no way of releasing or expressing them. Little did I know; that was about to change, although this would ultimately lead me to so many dark parts of life and recesses within myself that not only would I break beyond what I perceived to be my own limits and capabilities, but I would plunge myself much further into the abyss of darkness and totally batter myself, physically, mentally and spiritually.

I was in Braintree in Essex one afternoon in 1997 when I bumped into a friend/associate who I had not seen in a few years. We got chatting and after a while I was asked round to his house for a coffee, to which I agreed as it was refreshing to chat to someone I had known for a while.

My friend, his wife and I chatted for a while, drinking coffee and reminiscing on days gone by, then after a while a roll of tin foil was brought, pieces of which were folded and shaped. I was intrigued and it was made clear to me that heroin was going to be smoked.

As I watched, my friend and his wife put a tube shaped from foil in their mouths, put the powdered heroin on the foil and gently heated it from underneath with a lighter. This turns the powder into a dark brown/black liquid which slowly runs around the foil and vapours are given off, which is what is inhaled through the tube. This is also known as 'chasing the dragon.'

I was passed a tube which I put into my mouth whilst my friend held the foil underneath and slowly heated it whilst I inhaled. This went on for a few minutes and as well as enjoying the taste, which I can only liken to being a bittersweet earthy taste; the wafts of vapour had an aroma similar to slightly scorched candyfloss. This whole ritual, the preparation, the smell and taste became quite hypnotic. Watching the black blob of heroin slowly move around the foil directly underneath the foil tube which I was inhaling the vapours through, then once the heat is removed, the heroin solidifies.

I eventually had to make a quick dash to the toilet where I projectile vomited for what seemed like an age and

I remember distinctly the feeling of being cleansed as I retched and was sick. After a while I went back to join my friend and his wife, although I just sat there and, after around ten minutes, I fell asleep and dreamt the most lucid, vivid and comforting dreams.

I cannot remember how long I slept for, but when I awoke I was made a coffee, which I willingly drank and I remember sensations of total bliss and warmth surging through and over me. Total euphoria, inner peace, calm and serenity ensued.

I had £100 on me and it wasn't long until I was asking if I could buy some. So, phone calls were made, I handed over my money to my friend and shortly afterwards someone knocked on his front door. He answered and came back and gave me what seemed liked loads of heroin in comparison to the amount I had seen burning slowly on the foil earlier on.

I didn't leave my friends for around three days, just stayed there drinking coffee, chatting and constantly smoking heroin. Little did I know that, after this time, my world and life would never be the same again.

The Heroin Years,
All Eleven of Them

I vividly remember every day being fuelled by heroin at this time. Money was not a problem and, apart from the circle of people I smoked it with increasing, each day was the same and the feelings of euphoria remained. It was like being in the most comfortable stasis ever and the only comparison I will liken the senses and emotive states I felt are to that of being in the mother's womb. That would be the only place where we are totally oblivious to the world around us and in such a relaxed and content state that nothing matters. That's exactly how I felt and, for the first time in many years, my constant nagging and monkey chattering mind stopped with the incessant thoughts, words and basically the white noise that had been in my head since I was a young child.

After three to four months of this routine and as we reached the end of summer and the autumnal months started creeping in, I woke up one morning and realised that I had a huge problem. I had no money, my body was dripping with cold sweat, I was feeling sick, my whole body ached, I had diarrhoea, was shaking and I knew I was in the early stages of a full-blown heroin withdrawal (rattling, going into cold turkey). My body and mind had transformed into that of a heroin addict, basically I was in big trouble and I urgently needed to score and obtain some more heroin.

Upon reflection, it is easy to see how the desperation of feeling so sick and ill becomes the controlling force in your life. A sickness like no other and the only focus is to not get into that state, therefore you do your best to constantly maintain yourself, keep some heroin in easy reach and stave off the looming feelings of entering the vile and debilitating cold turkey stasis.

The life of a heroin addict is not a life, but a mere existence on the peripherals of society. You are entrenched totally and constantly in the thought processes of obtaining heroin and taking it. Basically, that is your life, nothing nor anybody is of any significance, except the longing and lusting after the drug, that's the whole of your existence, anything else literally falls by the wayside.

It wasn't long until I had reached the point where shoplifting became a necessity, simply to fund the habit that I had found myself with. Being disqualified from driving didn't faze me as the urge to stay well was my only focus.

Anybody who has been afflicted by, and succumbed to, an addiction will know exactly what I mean when I say that the addiction, although negative, ultimately becomes what propels and drives you onward, everything else is just superfluous and totally insignificant.

Shoplifting is seen as a victimless crime, I justified myself doing this as all the larger and mainstream high street shops were fully insured against losses, so it was ok, that's how blinkered my mindset had become. In all the years I was a shoplifter, not once did I take anything from small and individually run shops or small businesses. Even though in a drug fuelled haze, I avoided them and only concentrated on the larger shops and supermarkets.

Driving, although illegal, became essential. In essence, as a shoplifter you very soon get noticed, by the shop staff, local security guards and the ever-watching CCTV cameras that are seemingly everywhere, even more so when you are trying to avoid them and appear inconspicuous.

Travelling further and further afield to visit other towns where you are not known becomes like an excursion or day out and, although illegal, this essentially becomes like a full-time job. Early mornings would start fuelled by whatever heroin I had left over from the day before. This would get me up and dressed and into my car, then head off to wherever, then find a shop, enter, look around whilst checking for surveillance cameras, security guards and the Police. Then, when it felt ok (and in some cases, even when it didn't), I would grab whatever I could and make a swift exit.

As with any part of life, when you are in that lifestyle,

connections are soon made which then allow you to operate within a much wider area. It becomes easy to score and purchase heroin and, if that became problematic anywhere, I would seek out the local prostitutes as the majority of them, back then anyway, were addicts themselves and they were always accommodating and would soon obtain some heroin for me, along with some crack cocaine, which was another habit I was quickly developing.

In 1999 I received my first prison sentence and was sentenced to two months for driving whilst disqualified. Of this, I would serve half in prison, so I had one month to do.

Anybody who believes, falsely, that prison is a holiday camp has absolutely no idea what it means to be confined for 23 hours a day in a cell that measures approximately 8ft by 8ft square. Yes there are televisions in them, and you have washing facilities and you get fed three times a day, but the frustration and total boredom though and being confined is no laughing matter.

In 1999, I had been a heroin addict for 2 years and this prison sentence was the very worst cold turkey or rattle I had endured in that time. Sweating profusely, going hot then cold, vomiting, shaking, retching, chronic diarrhoea, not sleeping at all, my bones ached and the constant twitches were just an absolute nightmare and were a constant for around 2 weeks and even after that, they don't go, they just become manageable.

The first two weeks of my first prison sentence seemed like the longest two weeks of my life with the constant aches, pains, sickness and insomnia. I didn't eat or drink and, considering that by this time due to a two year addiction I only weighed around eight stone in weight, which at 6ft 4ins tall is not good, this time was incredibly tough.

After two weeks I was moved from Chelmsford Prison to Wayland Prison in Grisham, Norfolk, which was a category C prison, low risk basically, and it was here that I finished this prison sentence.

Wayland was much more relaxed than Chelmsford, a lot smaller in size and a much easier daily routine was set up and it was in here that I met Reg Kray before his death in 2000.

By the time of my release, a lot of the aches, pains and sickness had alleviated, although I still was not sleeping and, as I was to find out later on, the sleep pattern of a detoxing heroin addict can take several months to return, once (and if) they do manage to get totally clean.

On my release I quickly returned to taking heroin again, such was the burning desire to feel numb again and this, for me personally, is what it was ultimately about.

If hindsight was foresight we would all be exemplary humans and citizens of this earth. If that was the case though, we would not need to be having this human experience as divinity and alignment with creation and all that matters in this world and the very reason we are all here in the first place would have already been achieved. That's not the case though, and it is through our learning and personal development that we can grow and evolve.

Throughout all my life I had been seeking answers to my constant overworking mind. I had tried numerous ways to quench this. Due to being a young age and also being snubbed by many because of my constant searching and seeking,

I had turned inwards yet was ill equipped to find what I was longing for. Heroin, for the first time in my life, allowed me to switch off from thought, it gave me peace, comfort and staved off the incessant chatter within my mind. It has taken me many years of plausible and deep soul searching to realise this. What matters is that I have realised this and am now at peace with who and what I am, and I have no regrets whatsoever.

My stay in prison had done nothing to alleviate my urge for the blanket of heroin which I sought, like a comfort blanket or special toy that a child has to help them feel safe and secure. That is what heroin had become to me, my safe place far away from the melee and madness of this world and the madness within my own head. Although, in reality I had another driving whilst disqualified charge to answer to and within three weeks of my release from Wayland Prison I attended Court again. This time I was sentenced to four months in prison, so I found myself back in Chelmsford Prison once again.

I was already beginning to feel the effects of detoxing as I was admitted into Chelmsford Prison that evening. Back then, they didn't administer anything to help you at all, so that night back in prison was absolute hell with all the physical withdrawals of cold turkey and this time I would be serving four months, of which I would actually serve two.

After a really rough night which seemed to last an eternity, I was feeling really ill, angry and very frustrated with the situation I found myself in, even though it was my own fault and I had nobody else to blame except myself.

I could hear jangling keys walking about outside my cell door, which is an indication that another day is just about to start inside the confinement and walls of a prison, so I knew the time was around 8am.

I lethargically and wearily prised myself off from the top bunk bed and made a coffee, not that I was going to drink it, as the full-blown rattle I was experiencing meant I couldn't stomach anything, although just the going through the motions of making a coffee gave me a sense of some normality and that's what matters in prison, as everything else is so out of sync from the perceived normal world outside that to have even a fleeting sense of normal life instils a boost within you.

I was sitting back up on the top bunk, there was nobody underneath me as admissions into Chelmsford Prison the previous evening had been relatively minimal, so at least I could be ill without sharing a cell with someone else, which is never good or ideal.

As I sat there counting the bricks that made up the stark cold walls of the cell I was in, I heard keys outside and suddenly the door swung open. Standing there was a shortish bespectacled man clothed in a black tunic, a man of the cloth, and with no greeting he just blurted out, "God loves you."

I wasn't in the mood at all and without thinking I threw my coffee over him, I will never forget the startled look on his face. By now the coffee was stone cold although that mattered not as he pressed the alarm on the wall which instantly sounded along the corridor outside. Within seconds, three prison wardens, or screws as they are known in prison, charged into my cell and unceremoniously dragged me off of my top bunk perch and forced me onto the floor, which didn't take much effort on their behalf as I was so ill I was as weak as a kitten.

I was half dragged, and half frog marched along several corridors to a different section or wing of the prison and placed in what is known as a holding cell.

After what seemed like an age, I was told that due to my behaviour towards the Vicar, I would be shipped out to another prison, although no further action than that would be taken, which was a relief. For this slight misdemeanour I was to be taken to Belmarsh Prison in London which, at the time, was a category A prison and was the most secure prison in Europe.

I vividly remember parts of the journey to London, in a Group 4 prisoner van where the tiny compartments you are secured in are hardly big enough to sit down in and feeling as rough as I did, all I wanted to do was lay down. I felt totally lost and really could not fully comprehend what was going on in my life. Once again, anger, frustration, bewilderment and sadness filled my very being along with the chronic pains and discomfort of my body being totally empty and devoid of heroin.

Going into prison became a sort of 'normal' in my life. As sad as that sounds and may seem, it did. Between the years of 1999 –2006 I served nine different prison sentences, all for shoplifting and/or driving whilst disqualified. The shortest being one month and the longest sentence was five months. Regardless of what you may think, or people might say, one night of having your liberty taken away is long enough, no question about that at all.

The Cost to
My Health

There was ultimately, and always going to be, serious threats to my own health living the way that I was. With all the years of self-abuse, which addiction is, the price we pay can often be extremely high, and sadly and all too often, the price can be that of losing a life. I know I am extremely lucky and very blessed to still be here and living my best life to date. I have witnessed several associates over those heroin years die from overdoses and have been in close proximity with some, even present in the same room as the life force has ebbed away from them. I will never forget them and may they R.I.P.

As an addict, and an extreme one, my weight almost halved and at the height, or depth of my heroin and crack cocaine addiction my weight fell down to around eight stone, which is nothing and I must have looked like death itself.

I suffered two heart attacks whilst an addict and another one just after I got myself clean, so by the age of 40 years old I had had three heart attacks. I was hospitalised for each one and given various medications but I soon discharged myself from hospital at the earliest opportunity with the first two, such was my inner urge for heroin that nothing else mattered, not even my own health, such is the draw and urge to take this drug that everything else has no meaning to you.

My addiction lasted from 1997–2008, a total of eleven years and whilst I smoked heroin and crack cocaine a lot of the time, I started injecting in 2000 and for the next eight years until I quit, I have injected in my arms, legs, neck, feet, hands and groin. After all this prolific and constant abuse upon my body, it really is a wonder I am here at all. Yet here I am and I am so proud to be sharing my story with you all and in doing so, if my words and experiences can reach, touch, comfort and maybe inspire others to avoid the pitfalls that I have fallen into and been totally consumed by, then all that I have been through has been worth it.

In 2007 I woke up one morning and felt as if I was being strangled, I was literally gasping for breath and felt absolutely terrible. I tentatively shuffled to the bathroom and, as I could hardly breathe and was struggling for air, I looked in the bathroom mirror and was astounded to see my head was double the usual size and looked as if it had been pumped up like a football. I knew something was seriously wrong, so

I managed to contact a neighbour who called an ambulance for me and as I waited I cooked up a large hit of heroin and injected it in the hope that it would sustain me whilst I was taken to hospital.

I was stretchered out into the ambulance and taken, with the lights and sirens on, straight to Colchester General Hospital. Visiting there seemed to be becoming a theme in my life. I absolutely dread hospitals; the clinical stench, the coldness of them and the awareness of sick and very ill people makes them by no means inviting, yet a necessity. We are extremely lucky to have our NHS and I just hope that those in power don't end up destroying this much needed and essential service for those who need it the most.

I remember that as soon as I arrived at Colchester Hospital, there were several doctors and various other medical staff attending to me as I remained on the trolley. I was having my temperature taken, various injections and tubes were put into my arm and linked up to a drip and within what seemed a matter of a few minutes, I began feeling extremely drowsy, a mixture of the heroin I had injected earlier and the pharmaceutical drugs I was having intravenously administered by the drip stand above my head.

I remember being told I was going to be taken by ambulance to Ipswich Hospital for an emergency operation. Apart from that, and vaguely coming round slightly mid journey where I remember feeling sick as the blue lights on the roof of the ambulance penetrated my semi-conscious state and made me feel incredibly nauseous, I remember nothing else and still was not sure as to what was wrong with me.

The next thing I remember was having lights shone into my eyes and being spoken to by what seemed like many different voices from several people. A totally confusing time indeed and for the medics attending me it would have been blatantly obvious that I was a heroin addict as signs of injecting were strewn across my body.

I remember focusing on one of the male doctor's faces as he came in close proximity to me and carefully explained that I had chronic septicaemia and did I agree to an emergency tracheotomy which, he told me, would save my life. So I verbally agreed and I remember no more until I came round on a ward much later.

My whole body was feeling violated, I was absolutely exhausted and my body and mind, my spirit as well, were feeling totally crushed and numb, right through to my very core.

As I slowly regained consciousness and fought to focus my eyes on my surroundings in this hospital ward and setting, a nurse came over to me and explained what had happened to me and the operational procedures I had undergone.

An emergency tracheotomy had been performed which allowed me to breathe as the septicaemia, or blood poisoning I had was very severe. They had removed ten of my lower teeth, removed some pieces of my lower jaw bone as the poison had turned it porous. Also, they had inserted two drainage tubes underneath my chin, one each side which allowed all the poison, blood and gunk to flow out.

This nurse also told me that they had prescribed me methadone, a heroin substitute, as it was obvious I was a heroin addict and as my body had gone through enough trauma due to the operation, my body did not need the added pressures of going into heroin withdrawal.

Due to the various drugs that had been administered during the operation, I had been out for the count for 72 hours. I kept drifting off for the next few days but at least I wasn't feeling the effects of withdrawal as the methadone they had prescribed was keeping me relatively comfortable, and staving off all the worst symptoms of heroin withdrawal.

I remained in Ipswich Hospital for over three weeks and slowly began to recuperate. I also started to eat properly for the first time in months, probably years, although this would prove to be short lived because as soon as I was discharged I immediately returned to taking heroin and crack cocaine once again.

The cost of addiction on my physical health was immense. I still carry many of the physical scars now, and will do for the rest of my life. Upon reflection, it really is totally absurd how much I systematically abused my body and all that I have inflicted upon it. Yet, as I have said before, I know I am one of the lucky ones and managed to ultimately break free from the vile chains of addiction and lived to tell the tale.

Addiction also took a massive toll on me mentally and spiritually. As I became a permanent slave to heroin, all rationality and other thoughts were eradicated as the base urge to survive and maintain my addiction became paramount and my only goal each day was to not go into the cold turkey state of withdrawal.

Everything else got pushed to the side and the dominant focus in my life was my urge and lust to earn money to buy the drugs. Then the actual purchasing, or scoring them, which at times could prove extremely tedious and very lengthy. Once I had the heroin and crack cocaine, it was often extremely tough to administer them into my body.

I have on numerous occasions tried for a couple of hours to find a vein in my body that would allow me to inject the drugs. Due to the abuse and high usage, often with blunt needles, my veins had collapsed, or if not fully collapsed, it was often extremely hard to find an area where I could inject into.

Personal hygiene became overlooked and ignored, as I did not have money to buy food, new clothes or even pay for household bills simply because as you chase and fund your addiction, everything else becomes surplus to requirements, the only focus becomes the drug.

Addiction is no way to live. Yes, there are functioning addicts, and also high-flying ones. I have known school teachers, nurses, solicitors and many other professional and highly respected members of the community who are addicts, yet nobody would ever know as in day to day life they function just fine and show no tell-tale signs of their darker side of life.

High drug use and prolonged dependency eradicates our inner essence. Our base traits, such as real love, compassion, empathy and reality, all become suppressed and skewed as the drug reaches inside of you and rips your heart and soul out, leaving you nothing but the intense longing for your drug of choice.

The knock-on effects of all of this combined upon our mental health and general wellbeing is, to say the least, extreme. So when you next become aware of someone who is suffering from an addiction, try to imagine the immense heartache and inner pain they are constantly feeling. They just suppress it, and are unable to address their problems at that point in time, so judge not and just know that by a cruel twist of fate, it could be you in their shoes.

Shot at Point Blank Range

In late 2006 I was living in a flat in Colchester, Essex. My heroin and crack cocaine addictions were massive and for the majority of the time I was, through shoplifting; earning well and funding my lifestyle. I was also managing to pay my utility bills, which is a huge bonus when you have an addiction that rules every waking moment of your life.

For the most part of this period I kept myself to myself and did my own thing, apart from when I needed to buy, or score some drugs. Then I would see other people and they would become aware of how much I was spending at a time. Jealousy is all too rife in this world and it can be condensed in the world of drugs and sadly people talk.

I remember it was a Saturday night and Match of the Day was on the TV. I was watching the highlights of that afternoon's Premier League football matches and was comfortably numb from a rather large injection of a cocktail of heroin and crack cocaine.

I heard a loud bang outside but didn't think anything of it as I lived in a small block of four flats. I just assumed it was one of the neighbours either going out or coming home.

Suddenly my front door was smashed open and this instantly brought me to my senses as when that had happened in the past it was due to a Police raid. I opened up the front room door which led into a small hallway where the front door was. Upon entering the hallway I was confronted by two masked people and one of them held a pistol to my head.

They shouted at me several times to hand over any drugs and money but I denied having any. The person forced the pistol to my forehead and told me he would shoot if I didn't hand over the goods.

The second person was in the front room trashing the place in the search for any money and drugs that they could find. There was none in the front room as I had taken it all, what I did have was safely hidden outside of my flat, so I genuinely didn't have anything in my flat.

Upon realising the place was empty, the one pushing the pistol at my head pulled the trigger and nothing happened. My body was frozen to the spot and to say I was a bit nervous is an understatement as all I knew was that being shot would surely hurt, especially at point blank range and in the head.

The person holding the gun squeezed the trigger again and the gun went off. This obviously worried them both as my head moved back from the pain and my face was covered in blood and I was bleeding profusely.

I was totally dazed and in a fluster, I had obviously gone into shock from it all. It is crazy how my mind was working as the first thing I did was to push the front door shut and secure it. I then went to the bathroom, still with blood dripping everywhere and to my surprise a huge egg sized lump was present. It was whilst touching the lump that I became aware that the gun had been a ball bearing gun and the first trigger pull had jammed, yet the second pull had shot two pellets straight into my head.

I used a pair of tweezers and dug out both pellets which were plastic, although I can assure you the gun looked real and the ferocity at which those ball bearings penetrated my forehead was frightening. I still carry the scar to this day as a permanent reminder of that night.

After a while I managed to stem the flow of blood and put a couple of plasters over the wound, which hurt like mad, as you would expect it to.

Once I had sorted my injury out, I tidied up the front room, put the kettle on and went and retrieved my stash of drugs from outside. I then sat down, drank coffee and cooked myself up a large hit of heroin and crack cocaine as, by then I was needing it.

Ever since I was a young child I have been fearless; there is not a lot that fazes me. It's strange really as I have no idea where this trait of dogged resilience stems from. All I can presume is that since birth I have been faced with adversities and trials, so I suppose it all becomes second nature to just dig deep and carry on.

There was absolutely no way that I was going to show fear to a couple of masked intruders, why should I?

It is a tough world when you step over the line and cross into the world where it literally is every man/woman for themselves. If I had buckled and handed over my drugs stash and all the money I had, this would have only given them carte blanche to return anytime they wanted a hit or some money.

I admit that looking down the barrel of a gun is not ideal, and I wouldn't wish that experience on anybody, although this was the world in which I was living, it's that simple.

Throughout the drug world of Colchester, this attempted and botched robbery on me made those who perpetrated it look like absolute morons and even though I ended up walking around with an egg size lump of an injury on my head for several weeks, I continued to do what I was doing without any repercussions from this experience.

There is an age old saying that there is a code of practice, and ethics, amongst criminals, which to some extent there is and I have met and spent time with several villains in my time. Some of them I have huge respect for as the integrity they show surpasses that of many so-called respectable people who live in the 'normal' society.

Within the very murky and shady world of drugs, once you cross over and become an addict, you are, for the most part of it, on your own as desperation takes over. It is then that it falls upon the individual to, hopefully, stick to and adhere to their own code of ethics and personal integrity. Sadly, as this experience shows, some people have no morals or scruples at all.

The Epiphany of Being Multiply Stabbed

In late summer of 2008 I was strolling with an associate and we were on our way to purchase some heroin and crack cocaine. I remember it so vividly, the Sun was shining, it was a peaceful day, and all was good in the world, or as good as it can be when you have a massive double addiction, or, if you throw methadone into the addiction mix I had, it was a triple dependency.

Little did I know what was about to happen as I walked along, minding my own business through the back streets of Colchester in Essex. For what was about to happen was to prove almost fatal, yet hindsight shows me that more often than not, through adversity, we are often gifted the chance to realise what this life is all about. From there the onus falls entirely upon us to act to create the much needed changes. So often our downfalls provide us with springboards and can be the catalyst to start becoming the best versions of ourselves.

In my drug fuelled haze I was oblivious to the sound of hurried footsteps coming from behind me, suddenly I was aware of being hit fairly hard three times in my left shoulder and upper back region. It turned out that I had been hurriedly robbed of the £1,500 I had in my back pocket, although this was the last thing on my mind at the time.

As I stood there feeling rather dazed, I reached around with my right hand onto my left shoulder and instantly felt dampness and recognised the warm and sticky feeling as being my own blood. I hadn't been punched; I had been stabbed three times.

Memory tells me that my body started going into shock, I remember looking at my friend/associate in total disbelief as I felt the blood oozing from my wounds, running down my back, soaking the whole left hand side of my body and seeping through my clothing.

I remember the feelings of complete disorientation and weakness emanating through every single cell and pore of my entire body. My friend looked at me in total horror and said, "Shit John, you're in trouble."

After collapsing and hitting the floor everything became extremely vague, almost as if I was asleep. Yet I was aware and, as I lay there in a semi-conscious state tasting ash and dirt on my tongue where I was face down in the dirt, I clearly felt and remember to this very day the life force leaving my body.

I will never forget the emotions, feelings and sensations that I was consumed and totally overwhelmed by whilst laying face down in the dirt that day. I felt warm, cold, tired, alive, oblivious yet alert and I cannot remember feeling afraid or fearful in any way. What I do remember is that I felt at ease, numb to the outer world, yet also aware of everything, comfortable and enveloped with a warmth like never before and even though I was drifting off and leaving this mortal coil, the prevailing thoughts in my mind and whole being were that of, 'there is more to life.'

The next memory I have is of being semi-conscious. Everything was a blur and I felt very small, fragile, totally vulnerable and as my eyes slowly became clear and could focus on my surroundings, I soon realised that I was laying down and in a hospital ward once again.

My mind was struggling to comprehend pretty much anything at this point and funnily enough, this sensation seemed to be a ruling, or guiding force and energy, maybe it was the cacophony of drugs that were present and coursing through my body, maybe I felt cheated from having lost all those sensations of euphoria which I had been experiencing whilst on the ground, who knows? What I do know is that that moment, and that awakening, would be my pivotal point and, in essence, my own epiphany.

Slowly, over the next few hours and days, I gained immense clarity; an inner strength like never before, as I gradually adjusted to my surroundings and the condition to which I found my physical, mental and spiritual self in. This time like no other would provide me with a springboard which would change not only me as an individual, but also how I saw others. The biggest lesson in all of this showed me to take not a single second of life, nor anybody for granted.

Awakening

> Rock bottom
> became the solid
> foundation on
> which I rebuilt my
> life

After my stay and life-saving treatment in hospital, something in my head had been activated, a switch had flicked and I knew from then that I would never take heroin, crack cocaine, or any other illicit street drugs ever again. Within two months of leaving hospital I had also become clean of the methadone habit, a synthetic and pharmaceutical drug prescribed to help alleviate and wean addicts from heroin.

With all that I had experienced over my life, this stabbing and very near loss of my own life was behind me and I now had an overwhelming feeling to change who and what I was.

This feeling was consuming me totally and it was this longing to change that kept me anchored and focused throughout the coming weeks, months and years. To this day it is the belief that the best is still to come that drives and inspires me daily.

As my recovery continued from all that had happened, I had to address my experiences and assimilate, recognise and work through them. In my mind, I could compartmentalise them all and appreciate my journey to who I now was.

To have been a long-term drug addict is not just about giving up the drug, the journey merely starts with that. Every aspect of an addict's life has to change, and I embarked upon a journey that was unlike any other.

Physically, my body was battered. Mentally, I was exhausted and so much so that to begin with I could only comprehend what I had been through and inflicted upon myself and others. I had no ideas at all as to what the future held and, in effect, my years of drug abuse had wiped out and eradicated who I was. I will make the analogy and comparison to that of a computer being reset to factory settings. I had absolutely no idea as to the tastes I liked, my colour preferences. I had no perception of anything really, yet slowly I began reprogramming my inner hard drive, piece by piece.

Over the coming years this would continue and, even to this day, I sometimes hear a song, remember a name, or get the waft of an aroma and these small sensations can rekindle a memory within me and transport me back to a time way before my addiction period and add another long and forgotten piece to the puzzle that is my life.

The recovery of an addict does not stop once they give up

taking their drug of choice, it is ongoing and a constant. They often have no friends or family left to support them. Many times they relocate to avoid all the triggers they recognise that played a part in their addiction journey. There is not a single aspect of life that is not, or does not become, affected by addiction.

My personal awakening was no different. Although I knew instantly that I would never take heroin again, the journey to rebuilding who I was and the direction I was heading was an extreme and arduous one. Although as I write this book now, I am proud of my journey and, if, through sharing my experiences and personal journey I can help, touch, comfort and inspire others, then I will take that every time and know that all I have been through has been worth it for the benefit of others.

I lost my dad in 2006. I was being held at Colchester Police Station at the time, for a driving whilst disqualified offence, so the news of his death was relayed to me through the cell door by a Police officer, not ideal at all and this just floored me totally, as it would anybody.

My mum, bless her heart, never turned her back on me and I cannot imagine the absolute heartache I caused her over the years. My one grace is that my mum saw me get clean and shake off the chains of addiction and, even though she never understood, she never let go and told me several times over the coming years that she was proud of how I had turned my life around. My mum passed away on 9 February 2015.

It is often in hard times that we genuinely learn to appreciate this life and all that it contains. It is ironic that I had to almost lose my own life in order to truly value it.

I self-inflicted incomprehensible amounts of abuse on my own body, shaking it to its core and pushing it way over any preconceived ideas as to how much physical abuse a body can take, without actually caring as to the damage I was causing. I can now say that I am one of the lucky ones, and I have no regrets at all, I'm just very glad and extremely blessed to still be here.

My personal awakening has imprinted upon me that every day is a gift, a new beginning and it is up to us as the individual to make it count and be the absolute best that we can be. This life is not easy; nobody ever said it would be. This is what makes it such a very special journey and along that journey we must take nobody, nor anything, for granted. For in the blink of an eye, our lives and the lives of others can be gone forever, cut short and be over.

An awakening, as I see it, is not over quickly but it is a constant. The further along this journey of life we go, our understanding and perceptions change. We see, feel and sense the world around us differently and this internally changes us and deepens how we view others and the world in which we live.

I can now see that, much like steppingstones or the fragmented pieces of a jigsaw puzzle, all of my life's experiences have all come together to create and shape me into who I am now. From this understanding I fundamentally know that this life we lead is mapped out for us way before we arrive upon this planet, and it is from this acceptance that we can rejoice, and celebrate, in the life we have.

From as far back as I can remember, my mind has been inquisitive and, like a seeker, I was constantly looking for answers. Although, more often than not, I was not equipped to understand how to find the answers that I sought.

Whilst I lay on the floor after being stabbed and left for dead, my consciousness altered way beyond any rationality I had and the immense peace that I felt in that moment between worlds would ultimately prove pivotal in forming and guiding me through the rest of my life. Immense clarity, inner vision and foresight had been gifted me and out of the darkest of times a beacon of light was imbued within me, giving me a heightened, and more astute, way of being; for this was my awakening.

Chemotherapy

It was during my stay in Ipswich Hospital in 2007 that I was told I had Hepatitis C type 1, the worst of hepatitis strains. It was no surprise really, although actually being told made it a bit daunting. I had shared needles with others, used old ones I had laying around, and this game of needle roulette had come back to haunt me.

After getting clean from my addiction in 2008, I was still at odds with ascertaining my whole life and all that had happened to me and it was during this period that I met a woman. Heroin addiction affects the libido and in all those eleven years of being addicted, sex only played a part twice and those liaisons were very brief to say the least. So to meet someone seemed, at the time, like a good idea.

2009 began and seemed to be all good. I was now free from addiction, living in a new area and was a married man. This was my second marriage as I had been married before this, although the first marriage ended with a divorce by the time I was 25 years old.

Life continued and a sense of so called 'normality' ensued. I started to find myself again, watched football and motor racing, listened to music, all of the things that are all too easily taken for granted. However, to me, after having nothing in my life except drugs, shoplifting and prison sentences as the main focus, to do these simple things was extremely comforting indeed.

I returned to writing, something which I hadn't done since school. Admittedly I was writing mainly for myself at that time, although whether people see our words or not doesn't always matter, as to express ourselves in whichever genre we choose gives us satisfaction and is so cathartic because it allows us to make some form of sense of the feelings we have deep within us.

In the latter half of 2009 I was given an opportunity to possibly undergo treatment for the Hepatitis C liver disease which I had contracted.

I had various meetings with doctors and specialist Hep C nurses to see if I met the criteria needed to maybe begin treatment. These meetings were often extremely intense and I had regular blood tests to monitor the damage to my liver and also to see if I was keeping clean of heroin, crack cocaine and other illicit street drugs. This had to be proven as, basically, they didn't want to waste their time giving me treatment if I was still using.

Eventually I was accepted and was told that I could have the treatment if I chose it. I was warned that it would not be an easy treatment as it was chemotherapy and, if I went ahead with it, I would be on it for 48 weeks.

The treatment I was to undergo has drastically changed since I had it. The timescale has now been halved and the success rate is higher, and the treatment is nowhere near as invasive as it was back then.

Due to me having Hep C type 1, I was given around a 40% chance of the treatment being successful and that's if I stuck at it as, due to it being so debilitating, the majority of people gave up and walked away from it.

My body had been battered over the years and to be honest I was in two minds as to whether or not to inflict more suffering upon myself. This was at a time when I was totally readjusting to life and slowly beginning to discover who I actually was after all that had been taken from me due to the constant onslaught of abuse.

In late January of 2010 I started my chemotherapy treatment, and this began, ironically, in Ipswich Hospital in Suffolk, the very hospital where I had been told back in 2007 that I had contracted Hepatitis C.

My anchor and nurse during this period was a really beautiful soul and she was called Lynn. As time went on, she even gave me her personal number in case I needed to contact her. She really was one of life's genuine people and without her full support and backing; I would have given up the treatment many times over.

The first treatment I underwent was done under the

guidance of Lynn and involved me taking three different drugs orally and injecting myself in my stomach with a fourth drug. Due to the possible severity of the side effects, and because this treatment was still in its infancy when I began the course, I had to remain in the hospital for the afternoon whilst being closely monitored.

I had no adverse reactions, so to speak, although I felt like my body had been hit by an express train and chronic lethargy engulfed me and I just wanted to lie down. My tongue felt like a lead balloon in my mouth, I felt extremely sick and nauseous, had a pounding headache, shortness of breath and found swallowing hard. All of these were deemed as not adverse, so I was allowed to go home. My then wife drove us both home and I just sat there as the traffic whistled passed and held onto a weeks' worth of the chemotherapy drugs I was to take twice a day and then return to the hospital in a weeks' time.

As the days and weeks rolled by, my world was consumed with feeling sick constantly, taking chemotherapy medications twice a day, injecting myself in the stomach, or top of each leg once a week and being bed ridden, along with regular hospital visits for assessment and to collect a supply of drugs.

My one focus in all of this was that, by a very slim chance, the treatment would work and I would be cured from Hepatitis C type 1. I lived in hope and that was the goal I kept in my sights.

During these months of 2010, when I look back, I am amazed that I kept going. I was seriously ill, was vomiting several times a day, hardly ate any food and when I did it all tasted very metallic and vile. I was losing weight and felt so incapacitated and removed from the world around me.

I had been married for over a year and the one person who, I assumed, would help and support me was nothing more than a very distant stranger I was just sharing a space with. If I could have moved out and left my loveless marriage, I would have done, although feeling as ill as I did made it not possible. I knew things were not right, even in my pharmaceutical drug induced haze, I felt isolated and very alone.

The stark contrast of having battled to survive a stabbing, getting myself clean of heroin and crack cocaine in 2008, although only around two years before, seemed a total breeze in comparison to how I was feeling whilst consumed with the vile effects of the chemotherapy treatment I was now undergoing; an absolute living hell.

After a few months of the monotony of laying in bed most days, taking prescribed drugs, feeling terrible and very sick most of the time, it became a highlight of my world to go to Ipswich Hospital and chat with Lynn. By this time, I was going once a month just to have blood tests etc done and to see how I was feeling.

At around eight months of being on this medication, I was phoned by Lynn and asked to go in as an extra visit, which I did. After a chat, she let me know that I had now got chemically induced leukaemia, sadly one of the side effects of chemotherapy treatment. Lynn told me that she was considering stopping my treatment as I was suffering so much and the probability of me being cured of Hep C were exceedingly small indeed.

I trusted Lynn and on hearing this news, I broke down and cried, sobbed like a baby in fact, as I was raw from it all, extremely fragile, very vulnerable and I was totally broken, physically, mentally and spiritually.

It all became a bit vague after that, although I do remember pleading with Lynn, begging her almost, to not stop the treatment on me. I had come this far and only had around three months left and by then I would have been on this chemotherapy course of drugs for 48 weeks; eleven months.

Even though Lynn explained very carefully what was involved, and the fact that maybe the treatment should be halted to allow my body to have a rest and I could have it again at a later date, I knew and told her that there was absolutely no way, that if my treatment was stopped, I would never undergo this again; it was now or never.

Lynn really listened and there and then she agreed to not pull the treatment from me. I just had to go back to visiting her once a week for blood tests and a general health check, which I totally agreed to and so the chemotherapy continued.

The last few months of 2010 were, for me, horrendous, painful and a total struggle. I was utterly ravaged by the vile effects of the chemotherapy drugs and I was down in weight to around ten stone. I was consumed with emptiness, longing to be free of this living hell I was in and hoping above hope that the treatment I was going through would see me cured of Hepatitis C type 1.

Even in my darkest of times, of which there have been many, most of which I have created and am to blame for personally, I have always been able to dig deep and find the extra strength needed. Combined with tenacity and the stubbornness of being a Taurean, I have managed to rise up and face the challenges, meet them head on and overcome them and this has been a guiding force throughout my life.

2011 was a very mixed year. I suppose it was inevitably going to be really, especially when you consider all that I had been through, not only throughout my whole life but the years from 2006–2010 had been very extreme, like a fast track and condensed learning curve. What mattered though, was that I had made it through all of those tough times and, despite it all, I was just immensely happy to be alive, for in my heart I knew that life was not always going to be that way and would soon start to change for the better.

In January of 2011 I received a letter, and I knew instantly that this was from Ipswich Hospital and would contain my results which would let me know whether the chemotherapy treatment had been successful, or not. I didn't open the envelope straight away, I simply folded it in half and placed it I my trouser pocket to open later.

As my recovery from everything slowly continued, I found enjoyment in going out for short walks. I adored listening to the birdsong, watching the Sun rise and set and, for the first time that I can remember, I could actually taste the air that I was breathing in and was ultimately providing my life force.

I eventually found time away and clasped the hospital letter, which still remained unopened. I remember sitting there holding the letter in one hand whilst gently tapping it onto the palm of my left hand. So many of my hopes were contained within this unassuming yet official letter and I hoped above hope that the results would be in my favour. I felt that I had come so far to face all that had come my way, yet throughout all of those trials I had always found the strength and tenacity to rise up, overcome the hardships of life and move forwards. All of these thoughts and emotions were swirling around in my head as I quietly and silently tapped the envelope onto the palm of my hand.

In an instant I stopped tapping the envelope into my palm and hurriedly opened it. Then, with a deep breath, I read the contents. It all became a blur and made no sense at all to begin with, so I stopped, took a deep breath again and looked towards the bottom of the letter that showed a few numbers and percentages, then I gazed right at the bottom of the letter.

I was now negative for Hepatitis C type 1, the treatment had worked, had been a success and, although this meant I would always test positive for the antibodies of Hep C, I no longer had the virus. To say I was relieved would be an understatement and when tests are pending, once you receive them, they do not sink in straight away, that can take hours, weeks and even months. Again I had come through, dodged yet another curve-ball and now I could really start to get better, allow the healing process to begin and focus on what I genuinely wanted in this life.

I wasn't driving at this point, the original ban I had received for dangerous driving in 1995 had seen me banned under new legislations at the time which meant I would have to take my driving test again.

Due to being convicted on numerous occasions of driving whilst disqualified and having been sentenced to several prison sentences during my years of addiction, I needed to take my driving test again as this would give me my freedom back. I had now applied for my provisional licence and could drive, as long as I displayed the 'L' or learner plates which were required, as they are with any provisional licence holder.

New Beginnings

By now, my marriage was over and I was sitting at the computer one day just browsing through various classified listings online. This had become another form of escapism for me and seeing as my body was still recovering from all that I had inflicted upon it, I did not always have the energy to go out.

An image popped up from a listing and it was of a dog, a 3-legged sprocker (springer and cocker cross). There was another dog in the picture, but I couldn't make that one out. The listing had only just been placed and it was relatively local, so I phoned the number and arranged a visit.

On arrival, the 3-legged sprocker was extremely nervous, although a black Labrador would not leave me alone and was laying at my feet, fetching me his toys and constantly licking me. The man who lived there then mentioned that the Labrador was the other dog in the online listing and was also needing a home also, this dog was called Payton. He was two and a half years old, quite overweight and was obviously very fond of me, so I rescued him and within a week we were inseparable and I changed his name ever so slightly to save any confusion to him and called him Pagan.

Instantly we bonded and Pagan breathed new life into me and that was symbiotic, as we now both had each other. Everywhere I went, he was there with me and having him to take out for walks, talk to, stroke, cuddle up with and just be with gave me a new understanding of life and, for the first time in ages, I felt like I had a reason to live.

Having walked out of my marriage in late August 2012 with only the clothes I stood up in, I headed off to the south coast with Pagan for some serious reflection and recovery time. I was bewildered and in shock from all that had transpired over my life, all that I had put myself and others through and it was around this time that I started to suffer with survivors' guilt.

Over the years as an addict I had known, and on some occasions been in close proximity to, people who had overdosed and sadly died. As the years went by and clarity started, I questioned everything and all of my actions. How had I survived, and others hadn't? Why was it, when I was taking more than they were, that I not been the one to overdose and leave this earthly plane?

I grappled with these emotions for ages and even to this day I sometimes find myself struggling with the whole concept and injustice of it all. I know that, to a certain degree, I will always be besieged by these sensations from time to time and I accept that. I know that it will act as a permanent reminder as to how very lucky I have been, for which I am eternally grateful, and give thanks every day.

It was during this time that I took a day trip to Somerset. I absolutely loved the tranquillity there and felt at peace. I had been visiting Somerset since the late 80's so it held a special place in my heart.

A chance meeting with someone I knew saw me being offered a place to live in Somerset. It was a five acre smallholding where I would pay a minimal rent and be responsible for feeding and caring for the animals there. I would live on site in a large mobile home that had been made to look like a log cabin. I agreed and a date for me moving in was set for mid - October 2012.

I had managed to scrape together enough money to purchase a cheap campervan and it was late one cold October evening that Pagan and I arrived at our new home in Somerset. A new beginning and a whole new journey had now begun.

I was excited about this new start, although I will admit that I was slightly apprehensive about looking after so many animals as I had never done it before, yet I totally embraced this opportunity.

There was at any time, between 8–10 sheep, 3–5 pigs, around 200 chickens, several ducks and 6 geese. As for Christmas, I would also have 20 turkeys to raise for the forthcoming festivities as this was all part of the world in which I lived at the time.

It was during this time and the early months of living on the small holding that it became clear to me that my health was not that good. Due to having suffered heart attacks, all brought about by my massive heroin and crack cocaine addiction, I was taking tablets daily and was also relying on an angina spray and sublingual angina attack tablets, which I seemed to be becoming more dependent on.

I had had Pagan at my side for just over a year since he chose me. We had proved inseparable and were basically joined at the hip. We were never apart and he was at my side constantly, no matter what I was doing.

Only a few weeks after rescuing Pagan, all I can say is that he would at times, act weird and would, if I was standing up, gently, yet continually nuzzle me around my groin area. If I was asleep he would gently paw my face continually and lick my ear, yet there was never an obvious explanation as to why he would do this.

A lightbulb moment ensued, although it had taken me over a year to reach the conclusion that Pagan was alerting me to an impending angina attack. Once this dawned on me, I worked out that I had between three to five minutes to find a quiet space, sit down and take one of my angina medications.

This black Labrador that had insisted on being rescued by me, when I was looking to rescue a different dog, had ultimately saved me and he would continue to do this countless times over the coming years. Animals are not voiceless, as often thought of, it is us humans that are deaf to the words they show and speak to us.

This strengthened the bond that Pagan and I had

immeasurably and our relationship became much deeper, symbiotic and balanced. He had never been trained to do this, yet was acting entirely out of instinct and to this day as he lays at my feet whilst I am writing this book, as he has done so with my previous books also, I am humbled to have him in my life and am grateful every single day.

Smallholding life was enjoyable and as it was still relatively new for me, it was idyllic. The animals all needed feeding and cleaning out and this made up the bulk of my day. Plus, I would saw up wood to ensure the log burner would be fuelled through the colder months. I would often spend time sitting down in the various pens and enjoy time with the animals. Football with the pigs was always fun, they would run around chasing the ball, carry and burst it in their powerful jaws and just play together like children.

Another favourite was being in the large sheep field. This was big enough to throw a ball for Pagan, which he would run after and, in turn, all the sheep would run after him. Times like these were so special and will always hold a place in my heart. The total innocence and resilience of animals is nothing short of humbling, they each live in the moment and enjoy life for what it is, a rich gift and a blessing.

As with so many people, I was no different, in the sense that I had been bought up to eat meat. That's sadly the way things were and are to this day.

In my position of looking after and living on the smallholding, I collected the eggs from the chickens each day; consumed some myself and the rest were sold. I have also killed many animals myself for food; chickens, geese, ducks, the turkeys

I raised I have also killed, again, to consume or be sold for Christmas dinners.

One of the memories I have is of a female, or hen turkey. For those of you that are unaware of how turkeys are killed; they are placed in an inverted cone, this stops them flapping about, keeps their movement restricted and their heads hang out the bottom and narrow end of the cone. Electrodes are then put onto the side of their heads to stun them before their throats are slit. As I electrocuted this beautiful creature, she just gazed at me and slowly, her eyes dulled enough and, at that point, I slit her throat and watched her life force ebb away from her.

I have also loaded into trailers sheep and lambs, pigs and piglets and taken them to a slaughterhouse. The slaughter-house I used to take these animals to was a relatively small one in Somerset, so it was not a problem for me to wait with them. Once in the slaughterhouse, these animals are placed in a holding pen and I waited with them, still stroking and petting them, yet all the time trying to justify to myself that it was ok to have animals that I had raised killed.

When it was their turn, as they knew me and trusted me, they followed me as I led them to their deaths and committed, upon animals I pledged to love and care for, the ultimate betrayal.

I have watched as they kicked, thrashed about and screamed in panic as they were each electrocuted and had their throats slit.

Do not ever believe that anything good ever happens in a slaughterhouse, as that's what we are led to believe. Away from prying eyes and the falsehoods of deceit that will have you believing these precious souls hop, skip and jump to their deaths and are killed humanely.

The very word HUMANE is fabricated simply to make the consumerist public feel better about the dead animals they are purchasing in these pre-packed wrappings. Nothing humane ever happens in a slaughterhouse, or anywhere else that killing is committed. Quite simply, there is no humane way to take the life of a being that does not want to die.

Take it from me, I have been there, led my own animals onto the kill room floors and watched. I can tell you, if this were a horror film it would be banned instantly.

After each time of taking animals into the slaughterhouse, I would become totally numb, feel distraught at my actions. Then I would have to return a few days later and walk out carrying two or three big bags of amputated animal parts and the lifeless remains of the animals I had raised, cared for and led onto the kill room floors.

All of this was gnawing away at my very being, I knew this was not right, how could it be? I was raised to be kind to animals, to help them and not harm them. Yet all of this was playing out constantly in my mind and in my heart, my very essence and it was crippling and debilitating my very being and psyche.

As I thought about all of this, I could see the heavy duping and indoctrinations under which we are placed by our parents, peers and society as a whole. Be kind to animals they say, yet they serve you chopped up animal parts as part of a meal. It is nothing but hypocrisy, and the sooner the façade of why we need to eat animals to survive is shown, then the sooner we, as a race and a conscious collective unit, can move forward and confine these heinous crimes against humanity to the annals of history.

I found myself caught up in a total dichotomy; on the one hand my heart was screaming at me to stop doing this, yet my incessant monkey -chattering mind was convincing me that I needed to kill animals to ensure my health and longevity. What a totally crazy world we live in.

Without our past, we cannot acknowledge our future. All of this, along with the culmination of my whole life has shown me that I am accountable for my own actions, therefore I own it. I have no regrets about any aspects of my life, the way I see it is that to regret is to long for change. I cannot change any of it, but what I can do is learn from it and evolve from my experiences. In doing this, maybe I can reach, touch, comfort, maybe even inspire others to change and stop doing what they are doing and create a better life for themselves, and all others concerned.

The screams and faces of all the animals I have killed and have had killed are etched upon my soul forever more and I will never forget that one hen turkey who simply gazed at me as she died. Pagan was sat beside me whilst this was happening, and he was staring at me also. These animals know what is going on and the same life force that flows through us is prevalent within them. We really can learn so much from the animal kingdom, our shortfall is that we don't listen, we view ourselves as being above all other life and we falsely believe that we have dominion over them all. Unless we wake up and change the way we see and view the world around us, as a race, we will never achieve our true potential and will remain in a perpetual stasis where killing animals is seen as normal. Yet those who oppose it are deemed the extremists in all of this.

After almost two years of living on the smallholding, I was really affected by what I had seen and done and in mid-June 2014, Pagan and I left and moved to Glastonbury.

Soul Searching

For the first time in many years, I found myself having lots of time to reflect upon my life and all the experiences I had been through. This move was going to prove very cathartic, immensely cleansing for the soul and, for the first time in many years, I was not hampered by addiction and the constant humdrum of life itself.

It was as if I had now taken a back seat and, although the world was continuing in the same vein as it invariably does, I found myself merely a spectator; one who is intrinsically aware of all that happens, yet does not partake. For, apart from undertaking the usual mundane tasks like shopping, I was able to dissect every part of who and what I was. I mentally stripped apart all that I had endured, ascertained it all gradually, then grew from the lessons and then compartmentalised all of these thoughts and experiences.

Glastonbury in Somerset is nestled amongst some inspirational places of great historical significance and the landscapes and expanses of green are therapeutic and awe inspiring. So, Pagan and I spent many tranquil and happy times just walking around and absorbing all the beauty that is in abundance in this spectacular part of the South West of England.

I was now able to drive. Due to my addiction and being convicted numerous times for driving whilst disqualified, the original ban I received in 1995 (with the condition placed that I had to retake my driving test) had a length in total that amounted to eighteen years. This, of course, was not just one disqualification but many all combined together.

So it was that, in the early part of 2013, I took my driving test again, although this was the extended driving test as the courts had fixed. It was obvious that I would not be simply gifted a licence and, like all aspects of my life, I had to work hard for this. On the day I passed, with merits, and was told by the examiner that the extended practical driving test I had completed was in fact no different from the advanced driving test.

Another aspect of my life which I scrutinised whilst living in Glastonbury was that of the foods that I consumed. Due to the horrors I had personally inflicted upon animals that I had myself raised, plus leading others to their deaths in a slaughterhouse; I drastically reduced my meat intake, yet I ate more fish and continued drinking and using dairy products.

I started to become fairly insular during this period of my life and, as well as walking Pagan a lot, I began to read quite a bit; to help understand the human mind and try to come to terms with why people act the way they do. Also, reading books on spirituality and nature engrossed me a lot.

For the first time I could see my journey up to this point in time and within all of this I slowly started to get to grips with myself and face just who I was and, in doing so, I examined every single aspect of the whole journey which my life had taken and shaped me into who I was.

Wake Up Call

As 2015 began I found myself driving with regularity from Somerset to Essex as my mum, who was approaching 86 years of age, had been diagnosed with dementia, so I was visiting her every other week. My dad had passed away in 2006 and my mother, who had battled cancer twice over recent years, was in rapid decline with her health and living in a warden-controlled nursing home in Braintree, Essex.

Mum had only recently been clinically given the dementia diagnosis, yet it had become clear over the preceding eighteen months that this was more than likely what was happening to her. The one saving grace is that not once did she ever question who I was and never forgot my name, as many dementia sufferers do. This must be totally soul crushing for family and loved ones to witness such a decline in those that they love.

I will always cherish the times I spent with my mum, and after all that she had seen me go through over the years. She had lived to see me battle and overcome my inner demons and was aware that I was beginning to write quite a bit, mainly for magazines; online editions as well as paper versions. During one of the very last phone calls we had, she told me that she understood my path was my path and that she loved me and was immensely proud of all that I had faced, overcome and battled through.

My mum passed away in the early hours of February 9th 2015 and, even though I was at home in Somerset, the nursing home had phoned me shortly after midnight, explained that my mother was approaching the end and placed the phone next to my mum. She wasn't able to speak, yet as the life force ebbed away from her, I was able to hear her final and shallow breaths and heard the exact moment that she ceased to be.

A small funeral service just for family and close friends was organised and took place in late February at Bocking Crematorium, a small suburb just outside of Braintree and, even though I was unable to read the service on the day, I was proud to have written it and the non-religious funeral celebrant that read the service did an incredible job; spoke eloquently, clearly and also with great dignity and respect, of which I could ask no more.

My life living in Glastonbury continued in much the same way. I read a lot, was writing quite a bit, more for myself than anything else, in an attempt to purge my inner thoughts and feelings. This is incredibly cathartic and a way of cleansing and purging ourselves. Once we find an outlet for our hopes, dreams and experiences of life, they become so much easier to understand, simpler to comprehend on a deeper level and, from that point, we can move forward having assimilated and ascertained the lessons we need to learn.

As the middle of the year of 2015 approached, I had to visit Musgrove Park Hospital in Taunton for an echocardiogram. This was an appointment I had been aware of for a while as my health wasn't improving and I knew that something was serious wrong with my heart. I was now taking three – four prescribed medications a day for various heart-related conditions. The angina attacks were becoming more severe and Pagan, bless his heart, must have felt as if he was on constant alert as he was still nudging me, pawing and licking my face as he was sensing an attack coming on before I was aware of it, which gave me a few minutes to gather myself, take my angina spray, tablets, or both in preparation.

It was in June 2015 that I attended the hospital in Taunton to have the echocardiogram. As I lay there with the scanner externally being pushed around my chest, the lady doing the scan didn't have much to say at all, even though I kept asking questions, she never spoke or relayed what was going on with me.

After almost 45 minutes of being scanned, the door of the room opened and in walked three men in white coats, at that point I knew there was something seriously wrong with me. They all huddled around the echocardiogram machine looking at various graphs and reading printouts from the scanner. After what seemed an age, one of them asked me to get dressed and wait outside and I had literally only just sat down on one of the chairs in the cardiology department when I was called into a consultant's room.

There was no way that this consultant could embellish what was wrong with me. He did try, and I just asked him to be honest and open as to what the matter with me was. After breathing in air through his teeth, which is never a positive sign, he told me that my heart was so severely damaged that I didn't have a tomorrow and shouldn't be waking up each day.

To say I was stunned by this is an understatement and, for once, this news left me speechless. I felt like I was in an alternative reality. Yet, as well as being the main focus of this, I also felt as if I was viewing it all from an external position. A very surreal moment indeed and I am sure that anybody who has been told they are seriously ill, and that basically their time on this earth is about to end, can relate to and understand the enormity of the situation.

In all honesty, the impact of this did not sink in straight away, how could it? I was alive, functioning, living my life, yet being told I shouldn't be. I was told on that day that I was suffering with the following:

Left ventricular systolic dysfunction.
Left ventricular hypertrophy.
Hardening in main left heart vessel.
Ischemic heart disease.
Unstable angina.
Dilated aortic root.
Central and outer heart calcification (hardening of the heart).

Aortic regurgitation.
Aortic valve failure.
Mitral valve failure.

So, here I was and had, in effect, just been handed a death sentence by a cardiologist and chief consultant.

My brain went into total meltdown and, in all honesty, the severity of what I was told on that day didn't fully sink in for weeks, possibly months. I continued living my life, mainly on a form of autopilot really as I struggled daily to comprehend that even though I was still alive, I had it in writing that I shouldn't be.

The consultant had made contact with my local GP and I had to attend virtually straight way, where I was told again the cold stark truth of the very fact that I should not be alive and was totally defying the odds when I woke up each morning.

The various medications I was taking were changed quite a bit and the total now rose to nine prescribed medications which I was taking twice daily. Regular blood tests were taken, and I attended Musgrove Park Hospital with regularity to undergo more echocardiograms. Even though all of this really played havoc with not only my physical health but the impact upon my mental health was immense as I was battling constantly with the very fact that, even though I was alive, the evidence was in abundance as to the fact that I really shouldn't be. It was a totally horrendous, extremely draining and very tough time indeed.

It's funny really as all of this time where I was literally just going through the motions of everyday living and even though

I was walking hand in hand with the shadow of death looming over me, I knew that deep down I would, as I always had in tough situations before, regain my clarity at some point and from that I would work it all out and be able to understand it more intrinsically.

I distinctly remember it was five weeks to the day from when I sat in Taunton Hospital and received the news that I shouldn't be waking up, to the time I had yet another awakening and moment of epiphany.

I woke up in the morning and, for the first time in what seemed like ages, I felt content and as if a massive weight had been lifted from, not only my shoulders, but my very being. The switch had finally been triggered in my head. I had internally been analysing all of the information stored and now it had been compartmentalised and I could finally get to grips with what lay ahead. I was not going to lay down and blindly accept this, not a chance. I was going to do all I could to continue living and enjoying life.

Out of all the lessons in my life, of which there have been many, what I took from this time and these experiences has undoubtedly proven to be the most important of all and for that, I am eternally grateful, and give thanks every day.

Take Nothing for Granted

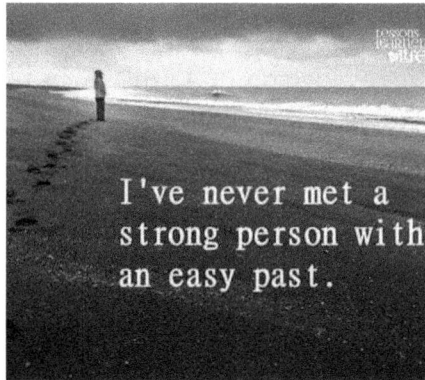

I've never met a strong person with an easy past.

We have but this one life. Everyone pledges to know and be aware of how very fragile this life is, yet until you have been faced directly with your own mortality, the realisation is not recognised and never can be. I would never wish any aspect of what I have been through and endured upon anyone, yet to understand that we should never take a moment of this life, another person nor any living being for granted, is a lesson that I do wish every person alive could somehow be taught.

None of us can comprehend a situation unless we have been faced with it, neither can we know how we would act and behave in any given moment, for we are all different and our levels of understanding and learning about life are never going to be the same.

With renewed vigour, a deeper insight into life and death and having processed what I had been told, I made the choice to become the best version of myself that I could be, to not waste a single moment of this very precious and fragile life, to not judge others and to see and sense the world around me without malice, without prejudice and to embrace it all lovingly and feelingly.

The substance of not only what I had just recently been told, but the many years leading up to this point began to dawn on me and none of it was subtle. I had perilously gambled time and time again with my own life, pushed my body way beyond the limits that a body should have to endure, yet I was solely responsible for all the abuse I had inflicted upon myself, nobody else. I hold myself personally accountable and totally responsible and once that point is reached, then it becomes abundantly clear and obvious that the only person who can turn it around is yourself.

I decided to write about my experiences of death and having stared it in the face myself on several occasions going right back from the moment I was born. I had worked for eighteen months at a funeral directors, I knew I was more than adequately equipped to tackle this often overlooked reality and very taboo subject.

I wrote a brief (around five thousand words) article about

how I viewed death, along with my experiences of it. Entwined with all the grief I had seen from families from the time I had worked in the funeral trade, along with what I had witnessed whilst working there, a pamphlet-style booklet called *Journey to the Summerlands* came into being and I self-published this via a sister company of Amazon.com

Albeit a fairly brief narrative of death, this sold fairly well, and was gratefully received. Many who purchased it took the time to contact me personally and thanked me for the immense comfort which my words had given them in their moments of grieving over the loss of their loved ones.

In September of 2015, I was in discussion with a publisher about enlarging my pamphlet-style book and the opportunity to become a fully published author. I jumped at the chance and distant memories flooded back from when I was aged seven years old and had stood in front of the class and proclaimed that, one day, I would write books and be an author. I worked intensely on this new book and in February of 2016, my first officially published book, *Summerlands – Pagan Death and Rebirth*, had its launch and was released around the world.

To have finally achieved what was, unbeknown to me, a lifetime dream of becoming an actual published author was, and still is (even more so with each book I have published) an incredible achievement and one that I am immensely proud of.

My thoughts, insights and personal experiences are held within the pages of each book and to have them on sale in every country around the world is incredible and truly humbling. At this point, I would like to say a HUGE thank you to my publisher and good friend Pete Gotto who set up Green Magic Publishing over twenty years ago. To have someone believe in your artwork, which writing is, is just mind blowing and for Pete to put his money where my words are, is absolutely amazing.

This life is full of ups and downs, we are all aware of that. Yet the dreams, goals and aspirations we harbour from childhood should never be forgotten, for we are the changes that we choose, and we can strive constantly to achieve these goals, manifest them and then make them into our reality.

I have experienced immense highs in my life, but on the flip side of that I have also suffered bone crunching lows and have sunk deeper into despair than most could ever imagine, none of this would I wish upon anybody. Within all of this though, I have had the mettle, the sheer dogged determination and the resilience to climb out of the mire which I, and I alone, put myself into.

We have choices in this life and as free-thinking individuals we are responsible for our own actions. It falls upon us to come out of whatever situation we may find ourselves in, stronger, wiser and more compassionate to all other beings and the world around us.

The roller coaster that is life will have peaks and troughs, that is all par for the course and is a culmination of this very intricate life which we all live and lead.

Life is not about voyeurism, it is about taking part and savouring all that there is to savour, although I have certainly savoured and totally tasted more than my fair share. In essence, I do not advise, nor recommend anybody to go to the extreme limits to which I have gone. In fact, totally the opposite as

I would like my experiences to help prevent others from living the sort of life I have lived.

This planet is a very beautiful place and living in the world we all live in today, there are infinite possibilities. If we set out to achieve something, even if we cannot achieve it straight away, that doesn't mean forget it and stop trying to achieve goals.

The intricacy of life is a very mixed bag indeed and sometimes situations occur to test us. Nothing is sent to crush us, just to instil strength for whatever lays ahead on this journey of life. It is up to each one of us to weather the storms, let the winds of life blow us around, allow the storms to crash upon us, then we carry on with determination and tenacity.

Each morning that I awake, I lay quietly and sense the world around me, I feel it lovingly and know that I have been gifted another chance at this wonderful and miraculous gift of life. For I know that whilst I am waking up, hearing the dawn chorus as the songbirds welcome in another day, that someone somewhere is losing their fight for life and it is this that ensures I take nothing, nor anybody for granted.

Hold onto Your Dreams and Never Give Up

Life teaches us many lessons, some good and some not so. What counts in the grand scheme of everything is how we prevail from our experiences. I can personally vouch that even the bad parts of our lives can propel us forward and can invariably provide us with great strength and integrity, and drive us onwards to become the change we wish to see in this world.

What is vital in all of this is to not become smothered by other people's perceptions of us and not allow ourselves to be negated by society's preconceived ideas as to who we are and what it is possible to achieve.

None of us know this road of life which we are walking, there are pitfalls strewn all over the place. It is often the case though that these trials are not meant to halt us in our quest, yet they are there to *make* us. Once we come to this realisation, then our lives become much easier, we feel much freer and from that point alone, we strive much harder to achieve our goals and ambitions.

If we allow ourselves to be affected by others' thoughts and what we are told, then I would never have turned my life around and I wouldn't still be here writing this book, and that's the truth.

Our lives don't always go the way we would like them to, that's ok though. We need to accept that what is happening is for us and not us. Once we live by this, our whole being takes on a different stance, one of acceptance and knowing that we are being guided by a power and source far greater than we are and will ultimately be led to doing what we are supposed to be doing.

Fear and guilt are the biggest and most detrimental factors that exist in this life. The sad fact is that we place these upon ourselves and that is nothing but counter-productive. In doing this, we restrict ourselves and that in itself is pointless and serves only to deny us our true goals and potential. We cannot change what has happened. We can, however, learn lessons from it. So, relinquish guilt and move forward with your journey. Often in life, the things we fear have already happened to us, so again, to be fearful of the unknown serves only to stifle us.

Once we break free of these two chains, then we can move forwards with peace, love and contentment within our hearts. We know that everything is happening just as it should be as we carry on upon this beautiful journey of life.

For me to become a published author after all that I have been through should show that we must never let go of our dreams. We all suffer knockbacks. Life is not easy and nobody ever said it would be, but the acceptance and understanding that we are responsible for mastering the lessons we each need to learn is pivotal. Once we embrace this, then we can be the change we wish to see in this world and become the very best versions of ourselves that we can be. Whatever befalls us in this life, we need to know that all things pass and the Sun will shine again. Like the seasons come and go, so does the time for us to be who we need to be and do just what we need to do.

On a Mission

As 2016 began I was suffering a lot with angina attacks and having to use my spray and tablets with more frequency. The total lethargy I was feeling was overwhelming and many times just to take Pagan out was immensely tough and debilitating. Pagan was now working overtime in his raising awareness of an imminent angina attack and there is no doubt about it that this dog that I had rescued had gone on to save me time and time again.

I had been gifted a Shamanic course towards the latter part of 2015 and had spent the wintry months and early part of 2016 completing this course. I have to say; the sheer inner peace, higher level of comprehension and the total contentment that I felt studying this course and following it as an aspect in my life was very rewarding and it gave me much more insight, not just into myself, yet into the world around us.

With my first book having been published and released at the start of 2016, I also threw myself into creative writing and would, over the course of 2016, write another two books and have them both published.

I was battling constantly with my health and the dawning of the fact that I had two choices. I could have succumbed to the medical evidence and what I had been told, and I could have just rested constantly. In my mind, that would have meant admitting defeat, and I just could not do that. So, I made the choice to push myself, as much as I could, and adapt to do what I could do.

Even without the angina attacks, the discomfort and heaviness I constantly felt was horrible and I can only liken it to heavy bricks being ground together constantly within my chest area and location of my heart and it literally did feel just like that.

At this point in time, I was having far more bad days than I was good days, yet something within me burned brightly and even when I was in excruciating pain from all of this, an overriding force and inner strength would buck me into life, push me onwards and inspire me totally.

Around the springtime of 2016, I was gifted another course from some people I knew that owned and ran a hypnotherapy school and they kindly gave me the chance to become a fully qualified hypnotherapist.

Again, and as is my nature, I flung myself into this completely. Not because I wanted to practice hypnotherapy, but because I had always been interested in the finer workings of the human mind and psyche, so I saw this as a great way to learn more about this fascinating subject.

As well as studying at home, this course was hands-on, which was great, and I thoroughly enjoyed learning about this ancient art and craft. Coupled with my learning about Shamanism; these two courses combined have helped me immensely since and have both instilled within me greater knowledge, higher understanding and clarity of thought and deep contentment within myself. I finished this hypnotherapy course and got my diploma. Over the years that I have helped others, I have to say that I have personally found this so very rewarding and instrumental in me becoming who and what I am, and all that I do.

I was clearly a man on a mission in 2016, and that has been a mainstay of my whole life, for if something interests me, or gets my attention, I give my all and throw myself in to it totally. This can be seen right through the years of addiction and even before that. Whether good or bad, once I am in, I am in, and that is my focus and drive. Addiction is a negative, yet to have passion is a positive. The only difference is our own and other people's perceptions of it all. The urge within is the same, regardless of being good or bad, and the commitment is no different whatsoever.

My second book was called *Summer Solstice* and was published and released in late June of this year. This was just incredible and gave me such inner pleasure as I was now a fully published author with two books written and put out into the world.

My publisher then offered me a third book contract, which I accepted totally and was really honoured to have been asked to do yet another book. My passion and drive is obvious to see, for my third book, *Baby Naming Day*, was written and published in August of 2016. So all three of my fully published books had all been written and released within a twelve month window, this shows how inspired and driven I was.

As well as completing courses and writing books throughout this year, I had been reminiscing and reflecting on my time at the smallholding from 2012–2104. Many times, as well as remembering all the good and happy moments there, I had been deeply thinking about and reliving in my mind all of the horrors that I had been a part of and inflicted upon all the animals I had there. Yet I still professed to be an animal lover, I believed I was a kind person and I totally believed myself to be living a spiritual life.

I literally woke up one day and, as with all parts of my life, once I have undergone deep inner thought processes, a switch was thrown within my head and from that point, a huge awakening was reached. From that moment, my life changed and I strove much harder and embraced what I needed to be doing and threw myself into that aspect of life and living.

I went Vegan and pledged that I would begin to live this way of life. In all honesty, this has been one of the best decisions I have ever made. For to choose to live an ahimsa way of life, to decide to live as cruelty-free as is humanly possible and to not allow innocent animals to be systematically abused, exploited and slaughtered en masse is the way, as citizens of this earth, in which we should all be living.

With all that happened in 2016, I have to say that, for me personally, it was a monumental year. A very condensed and fast track year of learning, writing, achieving, but also a year of deep awakening within myself where I was to embark on the most incredible of journeys which would in turn, prove to be my saving grace.

Pagan and I moved in December of 2016 to South Somerset, into a bungalow which is nestled in amongst rolling hills and with breathtaking views of the stunning countryside around us. We still live here now.

Within our lives there can be times (often after periods of deep soul searching, trauma, deaths and times of hardship) where we are forced to face ourselves, as if we are looking into a mirror. These times can be immensely hard as, in effect, we have to strip down and remove each layer of who and what we are, then examine all the pieces of who we are, face them, learn from the lessons and then compartmentalise all we have been through and learnt, then carry on with life in a better way than we did before.

This was indeed one of those times for me, and the easiest thing to do would be to ignore it all, bury it and pretend it didn't happen. In doing this though, we lose out on so much and in fact by denying various parts of our lives, we are denying ourselves our truths and our life. From that stance, nothing gets resolved and we just end up with skeletons in the proverbial closet that never get aired or spoken about.

As I have said before, I have an enquiring mind and I enjoy dissecting every situation I come across. It's like a morbid fascination to some extent as I need to know what lies beyond and behind it all.

Many will know that to strip down our very being can be, and is often referred to as, a 'Dark night of the soul.' A time when we journey within ourselves and touch our very essence, by visiting our very core and inner being, for that is where our life force emanates from and the sacred place that holds our truth which makes us tick.

It is only when we know ourselves intimately that we can hope or stand any chance of knowing others. In the same vein, it is only once we love ourselves in an understanding way that we can genuinely love others.

As I spent time dissecting myself, which took quite a while, weeks in fact, I became aware of just how special this life really is and how extremely lucky I had been. Not just to have survived it all, yet to have been given all the trials that I had endured through my life.

Without these lessons, I would not be who and what I am today, and I am proud of my journey and how every single aspect has taught me vital lessons along the way.

This rich tapestry of life is made up of individual threads to which we can make the comparison to our lives. Each separate stitch can never show the whole picture, yet with our journey all combined, we can view much more of the whole picture and, whilst we are alive, we keep building upon the grand picture that tells our story and how far we have journeyed to now.

Researching, Writing and Making Changes

"PROTEIN IS MADE BY OUR BODIES WHEN WE CONSUME THE APPROPRIATE 9 ESSENTIAL AMINO ACIDS, ALL OF WHICH COME FROM PLANTS. THE ONLY REASON OTHER ANIMALS HAVE PROTEIN IN THEIR FLESH IS BECAUSE THEY ATE PLANTS. ESSENTIAL AMINO ACIDS THAT MAKE UP PROTEIN COME FROM PHOTOSYNTHESIS IN LEAVES. THE IDEA THAT WE NEED TO CONSUME DEAD ANIMALS TO ACCESS PROTEIN IS VERY MISLEADING TO SAY THE LEAST."

With new beginnings come changes and adapting to them. I embraced my new home and, for the first time since I was a child, I really felt a sense of being at home, at ease and that new beginnings were about to start.

As 2017 began I looked forward to the future with trepidation and excitement, much akin to how an innocent child views the world and I hadn't had these feelings or emotions for so long, which made it all rather surreal, yet extremely heightened.

There was still a massive stumbling block in my life, one that haunted me and overshadowed every waking moment and thought I had, and that was the cold stark truth that I shouldn't be waking up each day. Each morning and every night I begrudgingly went through the process of taking what was, in effect, life-saving medication and although I did take them, I was plagued by the very concept of taking them and I knew that there was a better way to live and I longed to not take them.

Pagan and I spent a lot of time exploring our new sur-roundings and around the new home we had just moved into. There are beautiful country lanes, vast expanses of open fields and stunning woodlands all around. I find that once out and about within nature and not in the confined restraints of wherever it is we live, nature heals us and we feel much freer and lighter. Deep feelings and sensations engulf us and we can truly connect with ourselves, who and what we are and the natural world around us. For me personally, nature really is the greatest of healers and inner peace can be found when away from the melee of life.

I was totally embracing Veganism at this point, trying various foods, drinks and doing my best to eliminate cruelty from my life, to the extent of what is humanly possible and achievable within our parameters.

It is very strange, but, one of the first things I realised about Veganism is that it is one of the greatest awakenings that we can have. Not only does it reveal and allow us to embrace all that is good in this world but it opens up a proverbial Pandora's Box and this shows us just how horrific and cruel the world really is and mirrors just how much the majority of people nonchalantly and without question, consume, buy, use and wear animals.

A brand new journey was beginning and basically going Vegan would see me, as it does with everybody, having to reprogram my whole mindset and dismiss the majority of what I had been told and thought I knew about health, sustainability, the environment and, most of all for me, it was how I perceived animals. I resented all of those years in which I had allowed cruelty and mass slaughter to be carried out in my name, plus I had committed the vile acts myself and taken lives that did not want to die and the fact that all life has the exact same right to be here as you and I do.

By the Summer of 2017 I was offered a fourth book contract from my publisher, the subject and title was *Ancestors*, and this is again something in which I threw myself into and I loved the researching to gain facts and other information. This book isn't about my ancestors, yet a couple are mentioned. This book is a metaphysical journey into how, as a race and species, we arrived upon this earth and our journey to now.

As well as researching and gradually compiling the content for my *Ancestors* book during 2017, I was heavily researching and cross-referencing articles that I had seen online about how dairy and meats are seriously detrimental to our own personal health. I found these facts alarming and also extremely disturbing. I am Vegan yet, as a movement,

Veganism collectively embraces all aspects of life and living. While it may not have all the answers to the world and daily problems which we face, it is a perfect place to start from. It ultimately stems from the stance of compassion and nobody can deny that, fundamentally, that is where our internal and heart based moral compass needs to begin from.

2018 began and I was so proud that, by February of this year, my fourth book was published and sent out into the wider world. Not only was I now a published author, I was now a multiple published author and I still smile about this and remember fondly the time, at seven years old, I stood in front of my class and proudly proclaimed that one day I would be an author and write books.

By now I was becoming totally engrossed in my research of many of the world's prolific plant-based doctors and their findings, discoveries and the medical evidence that is proving just how harmful the animal-based products really are to our health and wellbeing.

As the months of 2018 rolled by, I was researching the effects of the animal, agricultural and dairy industries upon the environment and it really is traumatic. Yet, most of this is kept hidden, blanketed away from the mainstream, although the evidence is there and now it cannot be denied.

In late summer 2018, I was asked if I would give a talk at a Vegan festival in Sheffield, which I did and I was really proud to have been asked. From this talk, I was booked for different venues, for another five talks in 2018, all of which were really well received and the feedback I had from each one was humbling.

It can often take us a while to realise and accept the gifts we naturally have. If we do accept and embrace them then we can not only help others, but help ourselves also and I believe that if more people would awaken to what they, as individuals, can bring to this world, then the world would be a much better place to live.

I was now embracing a gift which I had been told by many people over the years that I had, and that gift is of communication, whether that is via the written word, or the spoken word. I was now starting to fulfil this niche and I am so proud to write books for people to read and I am always humbled when asked to give a talk. The one thing I take from all of this is, if I can make someone think, show an alternative, offer hope and give comfort to others, then all that I am and have been through has been worth it.

I still hated that I was having to take prescribed medications in my pursuit of maintaining a certain level of health within myself, this really now was weighing heavily upon my mind. Not only was I giving talks and showing cruelty free alternatives to others, but I was taking a cacophony of medications which I knew would have invariably been tested on animals, and this is so wrong. We only have to look at the evidence and it becomes clear to see that 92% of all drugs tested on animals fail when prescribed for humans as our very genetic make-up and DNA is totally different. Testing on animals is deplorable, archaic and has to end.

Armed with all my findings and proven evidence from the various plant-based doctors I had been stringently and painstakingly researching, I felt able to change the way I was eating and, although I was Vegan, I now opted for a WFPB (whole foods plant-based) diet. I cut out the majority of processed foods I was consuming and started consuming more grains, rice, pastas, vegetables and fruits. I cut out alcohol, massively reduced my sugar intake and totally cut out oils from my diet. The research I had undertaken reaching this point was incredible and I totally believed that I could begin to at least slow down the heart ailments I had. In doing this, there was hope that I could live longer than I had been told numerous times by various GP's and consultants that I had seen since mid-2015 when they gave me no time at all.

2019 A Time to Talk

I have always had a passion for communication, whether that is the spoken, or the written word. I find it all very fascinating and, let's face it, without it we would get nowhere in life.

One of my Great Uncles was, during the nineteenth century, a prolific Baptist minister. Charles Haddon Spurgeon was, in his day, a gifted author, minister and public speaker who managed to pack out places with people who would travel for days just to catch a glimpse of him and hear his words. My mum always said I took after him in several aspects of my life.

When I was at school, primary and comprehensive, there were several occasions when I would be asked to stand up in front of the class and share a story or read one out loud from a book, so I guess speaking has always been within me.

Many times since my addiction I have been asked to visit groups and various venues and share my story of overcoming the darkness and how I survived all that I have. This is something I am passionate about as I genuinely believe if more people shared their hard times as well as their triumphs in life, this world would be a much better place to be in.

Having the ability to retain information helps a great deal when public speaking also. People often need to know stats, facts and alternatives, so knowing these helps immensely. Plus, when combined with real life and personal experiences, it all goes a long way in reaching and touching people.

When I was asked to give a talk at a Vegan festival in late summer of 2018, I jumped at the chance and travelled up to Sheffield to speak there. This was really well received and was to be the first of many Vegan events which I would speak and give talks at.

By early 2019, I was booked for 30 talks across England and Wales and by the time 2019 ended, I had given 55 talks at 51 different venues including the illustrious and legendary Anfield Road Stadium, home of Liverpool Football Club.

The year saw me travel a total of 20,000 miles and often give back to back talks on a weekend. This was a much heightened, extreme, intense and amazing time and I had the absolute pleasure of meeting so many inspirational people that have become lifelong friends.

Due to my own research that I am constantly doing, I am able to cover several different aspects of Veganism, from the stats on horrific animal cruelty that takes place constantly around the world, and the onslaught upon the marine life that inhabit our oceans. Plus as I can retain information, statistics and facts which show the devastation that is happening to the environment that we all live in. I can also quote and recommend proven human health facts from the inspirational plant-based doctors that I had been researching for months.

I also give talks on other subjects as well; my experiences with death, overcoming addiction and how it is vital to our wellbeing to stay positive in this life, not always easy I know, yet still an essential part of life.

I spent a lot of time away from home in 2019 and I have to say, I absolutely loved every moment of the year, which was in essence, a tour of England and Wales where I was blessed to be able to give many talks on a subject that had instilled itself within me. I had by no means planned for this to happen. This vocation as a public speaker had chosen me, which is often the case and, as with any and all aspects of my life, I gave it my absolute all and thoroughly enjoyed every moment.

Ever since childhood I have had an intensely enquiring mind and if a subject piques my interest, then I am in totally and wholeheartedly. This aspect of who and what I am can be clearly seen from my self-abusive and detrimental drug addiction issues, right through to my quest to show change to others and heal myself of heart disease and become medication free.

As well as visiting many places in 2019, meeting many beautiful souls, making lifelong friends and giving public talks, I was continuing with researching all that I could glean on reversing heart disease and other ailments which humans are besieged by and afflicted with in today's world.

This is where the comparison between addiction and passion can easily be seen as, for me, the research became my drug and the more I read, learnt and absorbed, the more I wanted and longed to learn. The difference now though, was that my addiction (a negative) was a total passion (a positive) and I longed and hungered to absorb and retain all the facts, stats and endorsed medical evidence that there were. A fire burned fiercely within me, for it became blatantly obvious that the only way a human can expect to live, and lead a clean and healthy life, has to begin with how we choose to fuel our bodies and this starts with the very foods and drinks which we consume.

I was still maintaining around a 95% WFPB diet. Yes, I was at times eating processed foods, minimal sugars and some oils, although this was with no regularity at all and I totally embraced this new found way of creating foods and totally loved the experience, I still continue with this today and have no doubt at all that I will always eat this way.

I was still taking many prescribed medications for the ten heart defects, disease and ailments that I had been clinically diagnosed with. This weighed heavily on my mind and, at times, totally negated my whole being.

On the plus side, even though I was being more active than I had been for several years, I felt relatively good and through-out the whole of 2019, Pagan only had to alert me twice that I was about to suffer an angina attack and both of these times were in the earlier part of the year. Undoubtedly, I was now beginning to feel the positive effects of being WFPB and this was only the beginning.

Ever since my visit to Taunton Hospital in mid-June 2015 where I was diagnosed as being in advanced heart failure, I had attended regular hospital and doctor's appointments where I was stringently tested and had various blood tests taken. This became a part of my life and even though I didn't enjoy it, I knew it was good that I was being checked thoroughly and taken care of, which I am eternally grateful for.

Since moving home in December 2016 and having to register with a different GP surgery, my new doctor was fantastic, and I cannot praise her highly enough. Whilst having the frequent blood tests which were to keep a constant check on my heart, because she knew I was Vegan she specifically asked for extra tests to be done on my blood samples so that we could both keep a check on other levels, such as Vitamins D3, B6, B2, B12, folic acid and iodine. These are a few of the areas where Vegans can be at risk of having low levels, or worse.

It became a running joke between us both that I was the healthiest unhealthy person that she had ever met. All of my extra blood tests to keep a check on the levels where a Vegan can start to show a lack, came back every single time as A+. Her only response to this was, "John, keep doing what you are doing." I saw this as a massive endorsement and that is exactly what I did; I carried on doing just what I was doing.

As 2019 drew to an end, in amongst the public talks which I was doing right up until the 22nd December, I had received a letter from the cardiology department at Taunton Hospital.

The letter stated that various tests I had been having over the last four years had all been overlayed together and there was now thought to be some negative changes to some of the heart conditions which I had. This really affected me heavily as it would anybody. I was plunged into a bit of a dark place around this time as I knew that I felt better than I had in ages. Yes I did still get extremely tired and had numerous periods when I was consumed by immense lethargy, which I put down to just being tired. Although my heart conditions were in the back of my mind, I did my best to not dwell upon them and allow them to come into my mainframe thought as that would only have served to restrict what I was doing.

I was asked to book an appointment with my local GP, and it was made clear in the letter that my options would be able to be discussed further from there.

Each time I phoned my surgery, no matter what it was about, they were always polite, courteous and very understanding. Also, due to the severity of the conditions I had, this meant that I never had to wait that long for an appointment. If one wasn't available the same day, it would, more often than not, be the next day. Again, I cannot praise the NHS here in the UK highly enough. Often understaffed, overworked and underpaid; at the times I have needed them, they have proven faultless in their duty of care for me and undoubtedly, on more than one occasion, they have literally saved my life, so a massive thank you to them all in what they do, often against the odds.

I attended the appointment with my GP and we had a very in-depth conversation about the damage to my heart and all the tests that had been done throughout the preceding years. This conversation was really not what I expected, nor wanted to hear.

Even though I had not had an echo-cardiogram heart scan taken in 2019, a compilation of results from previous years had been put together and three consultants at Taunton cardiology department had spent time deciding what avenues, and options, were available and the best course of treatment to take for my health.

My GP went into great detail and explained that I had two options. One of those was to carry on as I had been, even though their feelings were that I was now at an extremely high risk of my heart just giving up. They believed there was significant deterioration with some of my heart ailments and defects.

The second choice, and the one that they all recommended, was that, depending on results of an echo-cardiogram heart scan, which was booked for January 2020, open-heart surgery was the best prognosis. I was told that the open-heart surgery, even though an extremely high risk, could gift me longevity and alleviate the stresses upon my heart which various tests and scans had shown were happening. This procedure would involve removing my aortic root and inserting a prosthetic replacement. Also, whilst I was having that operation, they believed that replacement aortic and mitral valves would help also.

2019 had been an amazing year, I had excelled and I had savoured every moment, I felt better than I had in many years and was eating the best that I had ever eaten. Surely the medical profession were mistaken with this conclusion? They had to be.

As with all aspects of my life, I internalised everything that I had been told during this meeting and, as much as I didn't want to think about having open-heart surgery, I couldn't fully grasp the severity of it all straight away.

Another year, an amazing year, was now drawing to a close and I was looking forward to some quiet time which would allow me to gather myself, recharge and look forward to another year and that is what I put my mind to. No matter what the future held, I was still going to enjoy and cherish my life, not waste a single moment and just be grateful for waking up each morning. None of us know if we have a tomorrow. Today is a given, enjoy it for what it is and if we are blessed enough to wake up in the morning, then savour and embrace that, if and when, it comes.

2020 Vision

The beginning of 2020 saw me with mixed emotions. On the one hand I had total dread at the thought of having to undergo very complex, though potentially life-saving open-heart surgery. Whereas, on the other end of the spectrum, I was looking forward to giving more public talks and by mid-January I was already booked for 44 different events. So it was the latter that I put my energies into and concentrated upon.

With all the research I had been doing for a couple of years based around Vegan nutrition, over the Christmas period of 2019 I had enrolled into an online course as, with the accreditation and diploma a qualification could bring, this would mean that I could practice as a Vegan nutritionist.

In early January I received notification that I had successfully passed the course, gained accreditation; a recognised diploma and merits, so now I could further my talks and speak from a qualified nutritionist stance, yet another string to my bow and another achievement. I knew how much eating cleanly and healthily as a WFPB Vegan had helped me, now I could put all I knew into practice and help others and for me, that's what this life is all about.

It was a cold morning in January when I duly attended the appointment that was made for me at the cardiology department at Musgrove Park Hospital in Taunton. I didn't have particularly fond memories of this place. All the staff were great, no complaints there at all, yet memories of impending doom filled my whole being at the very thought of what was being talked about in regard to the open-heart surgery which I had been told was highly likely.

The echo-cardiogram only took ten minutes, and I was then told that I would be contacted about the results. This is never ideal because, try as we might to focus on the positives, that little seed of doubt does start to grow and then consumes our every thought, no matter how much we try to dismiss it. I climbed into my car after leaving the hospital, drove home and then took Pagan out for a nice long walk. This was a perfect release, for Pagan and I always enjoy going out, so to spend time together is beneficial for us both.

I didn't have to wait too long for the results as within only a few days I was phoned by my GP and was told that, after careful examination and having studied in depth all of my blood tests and various echo-cardiogram scans, the consultants have noted that some of my conditions; angina, atherosclerosis, solidification of my heart and the ischemic heart disease I had, were now showing signs of reversal. None of the other ailments and heart defects that I had were showing signs of further deterioration. So, as of January 2020, they made the decision that no heart surgery was needed at this point in time.

I remember the phone call as clearly as if it was yesterday. I went quiet, which is a very rare thing for me. I distinctly remember stuttering also, and then once I gathered my train of thought together, I asked her to repeat it, which she did. I had heard exactly what had been said, I just needed to hear it again, to underline, rubber stamp and endorse it for me.

Even though I couldn't fully comprehend all of this instantly, what I did know and embraced was that I had just received a massive reprieve and all of the studying I had been doing, and continue to do in relation to eating, had paid off. Undoubtedly, I had successfully managed to reverse some of my life-threatening heart conditions.

The huge weight that had been smothering me and affecting my very being, the very fact that in mid-2015 the medical profession had delivered me a death sentence and told me that I did not have a tomorrow, was now being lifted. The sheer elation that was now replacing the doom that shrouded me was absolutely beautiful and this gave me so much hope for the future.

This news triggered within me a knowing and longing to now go one step further. I made the decision to gradually wean myself off of all the prescribed pharmaceutical medications that I was taking twice daily and had been bound to for almost five years. I knew this would take a while. Medications are drugs, just legal ones; this doesn't make them any easier to come off of though. I felt intuitive enough with my body to do this, so another journey began.

My first talk of 2020 was in February in the town of Barnsley, which is in South Yorkshire. There was snow on the hills as I drove along the mountain roads that day, the Sun was shining brightly, and I was so proud to be on my way to give a talk at another Vegan festival. This time though, I was now a fully qualified Vegan nutritionist and had reversed my own heart disease through eliminating animal products and adopting a WFPB diet and Vegan way of life.

March of 2020, and the rest of this year could not have been envisaged. A pandemic known as the Corona Virus, or COVID-19, was now sweeping across the world and the devastation this brought was nothing short of being of biblical proportions.

The whole world entered a lockdown phase, and this would be repeated at different times in various countries and regions. The death toll from this was huge and the ramifications upon families, businesses and our whole way of life with which we had become accustomed to (which was now a distant memory) was immeasurable and the world started to seem a very surreal and insular place.

It is often within our darkest times that great inner strength and clarity become highly prevalent and this was indeed one of those times. There is nobody alive on this planet that was not affected by this pandemic in some way; many people were affected drastically and some more so than others.

A time of reflection ensued for man. Deep inner thoughts and soul searching became a mainstay within people. With so much time on your hands, what else is there to do?

As a race and as a species, we now need, more than ever, to look at how we see and treat others, not just humans, but animals also. Regardless of which species we belong to, each one of us has as much right to live our lives away from harm, cruelty and oppression as the next.

We have no need to confine animals to raise, artificially inseminate and intensively breed them for food. For in doing so, we are denying them the sunlight and natural lifespan with which we are all entitled to have and live.

With all the talks I was booked for having to be cancelled, or postponed, only to be cancelled eventually, a period of diversification was needed.

I was now being asked to give online talks, which I totally embraced and even though there was no physical interaction with people, these still went well and ironically these saw me reach a much wider audience than I had before, which was fantastic now I had such a powerful message to spread. Not only had I raised animals myself, killed many, taken animals onto the kill room floors of a slaughterhouse and watched as they were killed, I also have studied the impact that animal agriculture and the dairy industry have upon the environment and the world as a whole. I was now a fully qualified nutritionist and had reversed several of my heart defects. All in all, these are incredibly powerful messages on their own, yet once they are all put together, they become undeniable and cannot be dismissed.

Behind the scenes, I was still on a mission to become medication free and this was going really well. I was eliminating one tablet at a time, listening and being intuitive with how my body reacted, then adjusting accordingly if needed and not rushing it at all.

I eventually became medication free in July 2020 and it had taken me six months to gradually wean myself off of all the various heart medications I was taking.

This was massive boost for me. For now, not only had I managed to reverse my heart disease, but I was also totally med free and, in all honesty, I can say that I feel better now than I have done in over 25 years.

During the late summer and due to the UK relaxing some of its lockdown rules, I gave three talks. Two of these were at Vegan events and these were great. It was so refreshing to meet up with friends and be back in the physical world doing what I totally loved. I also gave an empowerment talk in Birmingham to a large group of employees that had hit low spots and were lacking motivation in their work. This went really well and the feedback I received afterwards was just incredible and very humbling.

If 2020 has taught us anything, it has shown us that nothing can be taken for granted. As much as it is hard to be in isolation, imagine what it is like for all of the intensively raised animals. They will get no reprieve at all and for the majority of them, the only daylight they will see is when they are loaded into a truck that will take them to their deaths at the slaughterhouses in abundance around the world.

We all now need, more than ever before, to look at the impact our actions are having upon this planet we all call home and all the other lives that we share this world with.

A transition is now needed where we sense and feel the world around us lovingly, with genuine kindness and compassion towards all other beings, regardless of colour, race, creed, gender and species.

I urge you to please look at how you can help create a better and more peaceful world. We all have but this one life and it is so important that we cherish it, that we do not take it, or any being for granted. Life is an incredibly special gift indeed and I know, more intrinsically than most, how precious it really is. I took everything for granted. I gambled with my own life numerous times, yet a higher force has kept me here and pushed me forwards to do what I do.

As 2020 draws to a close, I feel so privileged, for not only am I writing this book to share, yet I have been able to rise up again and again, often against the odds and in the face of adversity. If my words and experiences reach, touch, comfort or bring hope to others and maybe inspire them to make changes, then all that I am and have been through has been worth it.

Reversing my own Heart Disease

My life has been varied to say the least, a total catalogue of extremes, yet every single time I have carried on. Admittedly there have been many occasions when I haven't wanted to, but situations have come around that have helped me to find the strength to push on through.

Hindsight is a great resource to have and, once we reflect upon it, we can clearly see that life has led us to where and who we are now. Because of this, our journey becomes much clearer.

Often, we can find ourselves undertaking something and not being fully clear as to the reasons behind what we are doing, yet we carry on anyway.

I don't believe there are any coincidences in this life. My view is that there are synchronicities which are playing out constantly, for us and those around us, much like stepping stones. A leads to B and C and so on.

Armed with all the knowledge I had been painstakingly researching and studying concerning how the health benefits of a whole foods plant-based (WFPB) diet could help alleviate so many of the diseases and ailments. In many cases, reversal of illness was seen, studied and medically proven. It was now down to me to heal myself, or at least try to.

I made the decision to follow a WFPB diet. This was easy and as I was Vegan already, the only changes were to remove processed foods, oils, sugars and alcohol from my daily meal's routine.

I started blending juices made from fruits, nuts, seeds, berries and vegetables. Not only are these easy to do, but they also provide the body, when done correctly, with all the macronutrients and micronutrients needed to power our bodies through the day, or at least a good part of it.

I also started experimenting with various ways of cooking. Whereas before, and like most people, I was merely popping something into the oven to warm it up, which has its convenience benefits, but not if I was going to stand any chance of healing myself and reversing my own heart disease and other heart related ailments that I had.

I suppose really that WFPB is harkening back to the days of old and pretty much like, apart from the cuts of meat, dairy, eggs and other animal related products, it is cooking from scratch and actually planning and then preparing a meal.

I started eating a lot more fruit also and this is always going to be beneficial as there are so many vitamins in fruits. I also started experimenting with raw foods, which is exactly what it says, although I found a different take on this totally raw plan and one that I still adhere to to this day.

Cooking vegetables became like a science for me, rather than just placing them into a pan and boiling them until ready, I carefully simmered, or steamed them.

Foods are considered raw if the temperature they reach does not exceed 104–118 degrees Fahrenheit (40–48 degrees Centigrade.)

Heating vegetables in this way and being careful to not exceed the maximum temperature soon became a fine art. As well as being heated through and providing a good hearty meal, this process also makes them taste a lot better, creamier and allows our bodies to access more of the vital nutrients needed. Our digestive systems don't have to work so hard to

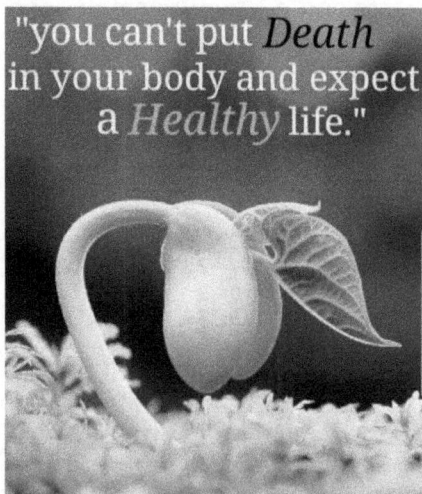

"you can't put *Death* in your body and expect a *Healthy* life."

break the partially cooked vegetables down, as opposed to totally raw, so it really is a much better way of cooking.

Removing oils from our diet is always going to be a massive positive, sadly they are placed into almost every product and we really do not need to be consuming vast amounts of saturated or hydrogenated fats and oils. We are not cars and we don't need all those to function.

I don't cook with oil and the only time I use it is when I make Vegan toad in the hole, and then it's only a smear around the inside of the dish to stop the batter sticking.

Healthy oils can be found in seeds, nuts and avocados, plus other sources, although this is my own preference as to obtaining the healthy oils I need. I have and have had this routine for around three years now. I have two or three walnuts a day and around four avocados a week and, knowing my body intimately and intuitively, this works simply fine with me.

Once I made the transition from 'normal' Vegan food consumption to a WFPB diet, the changes I felt started to happen almost immediately. I slowly started to gain more energy, plus with the exclusion of sugars, I wasn't suffering the highs, lows and crashes which sugar gives us. This is yet another highly addictive substance and again, it is added to almost all foods. We really do not need it, also it directly feeds cancer, so to cut it out completely, or at least cut back on it, will only ever prove beneficial.

I am still WFPB now and am now around 95% as occasionally I will have, what I call a little treat of a piece of cake, or a pie that will inevitably contain some oils, apart from that though I still enjoy and am thriving on the foods that I eat on a daily basis.

Becoming a qualified Vegan Nutritionist in January of 2020 was amazing and after all the studying I had done before this, combined with this qualification, meant that I could practice nutrition and help others, which I do very often.

Receiving the results from the echo-cardiogram back in early 2020 that showed that several of my heart ailments and complaints were showing signs of significant reversal and others showed no more deterioration was just mind numbing and mind blowing all at the same time.

Once we view all the facts and stats that there are around now, it does become clear to see that if we are willing to put in the time and effort, we can really help ourselves.

How can a body flourish when the foods we eat are proven to be detrimental to our very being?

I now see my body as a temple and, for me personally, I will now worship there and provide all the goodness needed to help sustain and power me through each day that I am blessed to have.

I am living proof that we really can heal ourselves and whilst it took a lot of energy and time to reach this point, it has been so worth it. Not only did I avoid having to undergo open-heart surgery, but I have also reversed several of my heart problems, then from there I have totally become medication free.

This turnaround is all down to me being Vegan and from that, I learnt other skills that introduced me to a much healthier and cleaner way of eating, that being WFPB. Now I am not just surviving, I am thriving and have honestly not felt this good in over 25 years.

Survivor, Plus Some Quirky Experiences

Having spent my entire life battling; against death, addictions, the establishment and those who attempt to subdue and govern us, I now consider myself to be a non-conformist conformist. Now this might seem like a bit of an oxymoron, but here is my take on it.

Having been fighting against what I always perceived as, and still do in some ways, an unjust society and regime, it has cost me dearly. Although I have no regrets, my life has been extreme in many ways and now, I much prefer an easier life.

I will pay my amenities and household bills, plus I pay my taxes and keep my vehicles insured and in doing so, this keeps the powers that be off my back. To a certain degree, I can come and go as I please without having to worry about being arrested at every turn. In this sense, I am a law-abiding citizen and entitled to live as freely as any other person.

What I do within, or outside of these peripherals, well, that is another story in itself as I am sure you get what I mean?

I was never going to bow down and roll over, not to anybody and, according to my mum, saying NO to me was just like daring me to do something. Any rules or regulations that were in place, you can guarantee I have broken them and pushed it to the limits each time. On many occasions, I have totally crossed over the boundaries of what is deemed acceptable and normal.

Such is life and in doing so, I have paid the price time and time again, often a very heavy price indeed, yet here I am and I am proud to still be here and able to openly share my story with you all.

I was at the height (or low, whichever way to see it) of my heroin and crack cocaine addiction at this time and, as Christmas Day fast approached, I was making money at every turn and spending it all on drugs. As I wanted a day off on this day, I was stashing loads of drugs away. I lived in a small block of four flats in Colchester at this time and in the basement there were a few storage rooms and along the ceiling ran all the water piping for the flats. It was in the lagging that I was keeping my stash of heroin and crack cocaine hidden. The way I saw it was, if it ever got found, I wouldn't have been responsible as it was a communal area. So it was here that I kept a substantial amount stashed most of the time.

Whilst it would have been blatantly obvious who it would have belonged to, that's only circumstantial evidence and would never have been enough to have gained a conviction on me, plus nobody else would have been to blame. The only outcome would have been that I would have lost a lot of drugs and cash and would have been ill from withdrawals for a while.

Christmas Day started off like any other day. I made a huge hit of heroin and injected it straight into my groin, which as an addict is the perfect way to start the day. I then made a mug of coffee and started smoking crack through a little glass pipe.

Laying on the sofa hazily watching the Christmas TV, I remember feeling a bit peckish. Food, when you have a heroin addiction, is not really something you think or focus on, such is the drive and urge to literally keep yourself intoxicated and high with either the heroin, or crack cocaine.

I ventured into the kitchen. I always had loads of sweets, which was about it, but lurking in the cupboards, which were almost totally bare, was half a stale loaf of white sliced Sunblest bread and a solitary tin of Kitekat cat food, which was a shock to me as I didn't have a cat. I know I would never have purchased that and it's still a total mystery to me to this day as to how and why that came to be there.

So it came to pass that on Christmas Day 2006, whilst totally out of my head on a cocktail of class A drugs, I consumed cat food sandwiches made with this obscure tin of cat food and stale white, sliced bread. I have to say, it was absolutely disgusting, yet I ate it all the same.

I still smile and laugh at many of these antics and strange situations I found myself in; it is pointless feeling any other way. All these pieces of my life have shaped who I am now, and I rather like me. Not in an egotistical or arrogant way, just the very fact that I have had bad life experiences and now I have turned it all around.

When I reflect upon my life that has passed, I do so in a fond way as I made the mistakes, yet it is I alone who got it back on track. Yes, I have had some lucky breaks, but it is still through my dogged determination and resilience that I have managed to crawl out from the pit of darkness and despair and learn from all the hurt and pain.

Contemplating my times of being homeless, sleeping on park benches, in sheds, bus stations and other random places has taught me to never, not for a single moment, take anything nor anybody for granted. Being destitute, broken and feeling totally worthless at times has now instilled within me an immense sense of compassion to others.

In these very trying times, none of us have any guarantees as to what will happen tomorrow, or even if we will be granted that new day. We all need to be kinder, to show compassion and have genuine empathy towards others, not just humans, but all life. Regardless of which species any being inhabits, no matter how small it may be, every single life is as valid and as precious as the next.

Another quirky tale is again when I lived in Colchester. One night it all came to light that I, along with a couple of others, had been the subject of a covert Police operation where they had been following us and monitoring us closely for around six months.

I can only imagine as to the vast cost of this and ultimately this expense would have invariably been picked up by the taxpayer, as in YOU.

I am in favour of having a Police Force. It's obvious that we need one, yet time and time again, they totally fail in their civil duty and it becomes like a personal vendetta against individuals. I have no doubt whatsoever that many people will agree with me on this.

It was one evening and I was in my flat in Colchester awaiting a large drop off of drugs, several thousand pounds worth in monetary value.

There were a couple of people with me and we were just waiting, chatting and looking forward to a big hit of heroin and crack cocaine. Suddenly the door came flying in and with all the shouting it soon became clear that it was the Police, which was a better option than masked invaders which had happened before.

This was a raid unlike any other that I had experienced in my property as these Police were the ARU (Armed Response Unit) and were all wearing helmets, full body armour and carrying rifles. Within a moment they had seized control and as there was about six of them in my fairly small front room, the place was tightly packed to say the least.

They were shouting and pointing their obviously loaded guns, mainly at me and I remember totally freezing as I became aware of several red dots upon my chest, these were emanating from the laser sights that these guns had.

To say I went from relaxed to being sombre and uncomfortable within a second is an understatement. These methods of confusion are made to catch you off guard and disorientate you and I can vouch that these methods totally work as I froze to the spot and am sure that I stopped breathing at the same time.

Whilst the three of us were being held at gunpoint in my front room, the plain clothes drug squad poured in like ants and it seemed as if there were dozens of them. They besieged every room in my flat, dismantled everything and had a sniffer dog running around at the same time.

I knew there was nothing actually on my person, nor in my flat. So on one hand I was massively relieved, whereas having red dots covering my chest was not an ideal situation at all. Plus, all the time I was being shouted at by these officers as the rest of them ran amok and trashed my whole flat.

Through the window, as I was being made to stand up and keep extremely still, I saw a Police motorbike pulling up outside and the officer jumped off the bike and made his way into my home.

This just got totally surreal for as this new arrival entered the front room where we were gathered, reached into a side holster and pulled out a pistol and started pointing it at me. At this point I let go and started laughing.

There we had a full SWAT team with loaded rifles, full body armour, all pointing big guns around with red dots coming from laser sights, then this late arrival pulled out what was probably the smallest gun I have ever seen in my life.

It looked like a toy gun and in fact looked less convincing than the ball bearing gun I had been shot in the head with before, plus this officer kept on shouting at me. By now I was sick of it all and all this commotion was out of order as I knew, unless they stitched me up and planted some drugs, there was nothing at all for them to find.

Ever since I was a child, if I am in trouble and getting shouted at, I have laughed. Not sure if it's nerves or what. The one time I really shouldn't have laughed though, was whilst loaded rifles were being pointed at my chest, but I could not help it. This didn't make matters any easier as now all the Police officers thought I was ridiculing them, so their shouting just got louder and harsher.

Slowly, the plain clothes drug squad kept reporting back to the armed officers that the place was clean and eventually, they had to reconstruct all that they had moved and taken apart. It was now that the ARU officers started relaxing and began to lower their rifles, therefore removing the red dots that had been seemingly peppering my chest.

After what seemed like an eternity, I began to breathe properly again and reluctantly, all the officers retreated and left, with the usual threats of "we will be back again," at which point I offered them a key to let themselves in, that never goes down too well, but so be it.

Feeling nervous that they might still be lurking about and also relieved that the shipment hadn't arrived whilst this was all going on, I walked around outside to check they had all gone, then made a phone call.

After hurriedly tidying up what mess the Police hadn't, more out of nerves than anything else, myself and the two people who had been with me left my flat, made a short trip to collect the stash which had now been left for me outside quite a way from my place, then went round to a friend's. From there, we enjoyed a night of total drug abuse and laughed about it all.

Looking back upon, not just this episode, but all of my life, it becomes clear to see that nothing much has really fazed me and, more often than not, I have laughed in the face of adversity time and time again.

We all live and lead our lives as best as we see fit. Massive pitfalls can often be strewn around, yet we decide how far into these we allow ourselves to go and then, from there, it is up to us to claw our way out of them.

As I write about several of my darkest times within these pages, I can clearly see and it all becomes apparent that I have, since birth, being playing with dice that were seemingly loaded against me and not working in my favour.

On the flip side of that, without all these hardships and trials, I would not be who and what I am today, for it is the culmination of all of the pieces of my life's journey and puzzle that have delivered me to this point in time.

I hope that through sharing my journey with you all, some of my life and experiences will resonate within you. Hopefully some parts will touch, comfort and may even inspire you.

For if that is the outcome, and within that I can deter others from making the same mistakes, then I am proud to have played my part and all that I have been through has been worth it and nothing I have endured has been in vain.

Much love to you all and thank you.

Shout-out to the Plant-based Doctors

Every once in a while, often within a lifetime, singular people, or a collective, come along and expose all that is wrong and corrupt within this world. Over the years there have been many people that, with their studies and depth of factual knowledge, have literally turned the world upside down as they show a better way to live.

There are way too many notable plant-based doctors for me to mention them all, here are a few though and if you research them, you will be literally humbled and inspired as to their discoveries, all of which are medically and scientifically proven.

All of these doctors and health workers can be easily researched online and all their findings and facts are there to see:

Dr Michael Greger

An American physician, public speaker and author.

Dr Greger is one of the world's leading lights in Vegan nutrition and you can see his studies and research at: nutritionfacts.org

A great advocate for WFPB (whole foods plant-based) living, he has proven that once transitioned onto a WFPB diet, heart disease starts to show signs of reversal in as little as three weeks. His studies are some of the most prolific and he has also helped to demonstrate that type 2 diabetes can be alleviated and totally reversed by adopting a WFPB diet.

T. Colin Campbell

Thomas Colin Campbell is an American biochemist, and his speciality is the effect of nutrition on long term health in humans.

He is notable for his advocacy of a low fat WFPB diet and his website is: nutritionstudies.org

He shows us and alerts us to the very fact that each one of us has the right to see and know the truths behind the very foods which we eat and how we can achieve better health by abstaining from the consumption of meats and dairy products.

Dr Caldwell Esselstyn

An American physician who has come up with, through his extensive studies and research, the revolutionary and scientifically proven nutrition-based cure that exponentially reverses heart disease.

He was a surgeon at the Cleveland Clinic for over 35 years and was treating breast cancer patients when he realised that he wasn't actually helping them and knew he could do much more for them via addressing the very foods that they were consuming.

He has also shown that, not only will plant-based diets stop heart disease; they can fully reverse it also.

Check out his findings and evidence at: dresselstyn.com

Angie Sadeghi, MD

A diplomat of the American board of gastroenterology, Dr Angie Sadeghi is undoubtedly one of, if not the leading light in her field.

Having cured her own chronic illnesses like eczema and fibromyalgia by going Vegan and adopting a WFPB diet, Angie is now an advocate for this way of life and runs her own private clinic in California where she treats patients for a wide range of ailments including digestive issues and illnesses related to the stomach, liver, oesophagus and colon.

Dr Sadeghi's website is: drangiehealth.com

Dean Ornish, MD

Dean Ornish is a well known advocate in the treatment of preventing heart disease and some types of cancer.

His work inspired and encouraged many other Vegan Dr's to pursue this path of treatment of patients by recommending that they follow a whole foods Vegan diet.

Dr Ornish's website is: deanornish.com

In our constant pursuit to gain health and longevity of life, due to societal and peer pressures, we have totally overlooked the one component which is staring us all in the face and that is the very foods that we consume regularly.

We cannot expect our bodies to run at pique and optimum performance whilst we are eating dead animals, dairy products, excess sugars, oils and heavily processed foods. That will never happen and we need to forget all that we have been told and thought we knew about healthy foods and start fuelling our bodies with clean foods that are free from animal products.

I am not just writing empty words here, I speak from personal experience all the way through this book and having totally turned my life around after staring death in the face several times, I cannot tell you how vital it is to start being healthy before you get ill.

I urge all of you to reconsider your place in this world, look around you and envisage the world you would like to see and be a part of and from there, make the changes needed that will inevitably ensure that the world we know now can be transformed into a better place to be, for all beings.

Medical Updates February 2021

Just before we went to print with this book, I attended Musgrove Park Hospital in Taunton in January 2021 for, what has become a yearly echocardiogram, which keeps a check on how my heart is functioning and, when overlayed on the previous year's scan, the consultant is able to see how my heart is doing and inform me from the comparison.

Attending hospital appointments can be a very nervy time indeed, for we put our lives in their hands and trust their decisions, where our health and well-being is concerned.

For several years now I have been swimming against the tide of modern medicine, as all the research I had done myself over a period of a few years showed me that there was undeniably a better way. Many of the diseases and ailments that humans are ravaged by, can be alleviated to a certain degree and reversed in many cases, as is the case with my own health problems.

Dr Sue Kenneally, who wrote the foreword for this book, points out that whilst modern medicine has its place, it doesn't always address the root cause of the problems and this is so absolutely true.

It has been a tumultuous journey to arrive where I am today, for I have had to go out on a limb and go against a lot of medical advice that has been offered and given to me by doctors, consultants and other health care workers. Yet now I know that my decisions have been correct.

Having reversed several of my heart conditions, I always felt that the three heart problems that I would not be able to help were the aortic and mitral valve problems and also the aortic root, which was narrowed.

The echocardiogram I had in January of 2021, has shown that my mitral valve is repairing, to such a degree, that it is no longer considered by my consultant to be of any worry and concern.

There is, in comparison to the 2020 heart scan, a very slight expanding of my aortic root, now this is miniscule and not visible to the naked eye, yet for me this is massive and endorses upon me personally, that through adopting a WFPB diet, we can, in many cases, although not all, heal ourselves through the foods we choose to fuel our bodies with.

My aortic valve is still showing some signs for concern, although in comparison to the first echo – cardiogram I had in mid-2015 when I was told I had no time left and should not be waking up in the morning, then I am ok with that as there are no signs of deterioration whatsoever.

As hard as it was to make the decision to look into how I could personally help my own ailments and, from that, to research and step into a world of alternative medicine, which I knew nothing about at all, was a huge step indeed.

This will be viewed as extreme by many and I have received, from some, much criticism for taking this stance and basically going against all that we are told about health and what keeps us healthy. Yet here I am and having reversed many of my own conditions and totally become medication free, I stand as a testament that we, in many cases, can cure, or at least help to alleviate many of the ailments that are sadly so rife in this world.

I have no doubt in my mind that the doctors and health practitioners of the future will be treating and prescribing life-giving foods to stave off disease and sickness, rather than pharmaceutical medications.

Disclaimer.

I am not medically trained and do not profess to be. I took the choice to become medication free through my own volition.

To reach this stage of my life, has by no means been easy and has taken me several years of hard work, personal studying, constant research and there have been massive risks to my own health, which I accept and take full and personal responsibility for.

I do not encourage anybody to wean themselves off of any prescribed medication unless they have consulted with their own doctor first of all and that they have their full backing and guidance in doing so.

John Awen.

Conclusion

Life is a gift, a very precious one indeed. Within that acceptance, the onus falls upon us as individuals to encompass all other beings into our thoughts, acknowledge their presence and honour the undeniable truth that the life force that runs through us and empowers us through each day and on our life's journey, is the very same force as it is in all beings.

Our role upon this planet has to be one of caretakers and guardians. For, as the predominant species in this world, it falls upon us to protect and care for those who are unable to care for themselves. We need to take the path of least resistance for all concerned and we need to ensure that, when our time comes to shuffle off and leave this earthly and mortal coil, we have done our best to leave this planet in a better state than when we arrived upon it.

The fact is that we know better and now is the time that we need to act and do better. Look around you now, the animals are being killed in their billions every year, the oceans are being ravaged of marine life and being poisoned by pollutants and toxins constantly. The forests and woodlands are being destroyed to make way for more intensive animal breeding facilities, roads and shopping centres.

We set aside more land to grow crops to feed animals than we set aside for human consumption, yet the meats and dairy products that are consumed are causing first world health problems, with the current Corona pandemic but also other ailments that plague human health nowadays. Yet still we call ourselves an evolved, intelligent and compassionate species; that's an epic fail there then.

Look at and consider every aspect of your daily life, how many animals have suffered for your foods, drinks, clothing, make up and all the numerous cleaning products you use daily?

We need to take a back seat, then realise that all life is equal and, in the grand scheme of it all, every being has a purpose. We each need to be able to live our lives and, in doing so, fulfil that purpose. With that, every single being is being beneficial to the whole and from there, we have a balanced ecosystem that will stand the test of time and ensure longevity for all involved.

Having personally experienced addiction, chemotherapy, being shot, stabbed, killing animals myself and watching as animals I had raised were slaughtered in front of me, being diagnosed with advanced heart failure, working incredibly hard to reverse heart disease within myself; I ask you to not be flippant with life.

I have no regrets at all and I know that my life has been incredibly challenging, yet I am so very lucky to have been gifted chance after chance and now, having experienced all that I have, I am able to speak about wrong doings, then about changing and becoming a better person for having lived the life that I have.

We are all here but for a short time, a fleeting glimpse in essence. Before we know it, our time will have gone, and we will leave this world. Before we do go, let us work together, for that is how we are supposed to be living.

In writing this book, I have had to face some very dark aspects of my life and in writing it all down for the world to see I have openly and candidly bared my soul to you all. I am honoured that you have read this book and I hope it has given you proverbial food for thought and that it will make you think about your life, your actions and input upon this planet and also think about making changes which will bring about less cruelty, a cleaner environment and better physical health for you.

Veganism may not have the answers to all of the world's problems, it sure is a great starting place though and once we all awaken to this concept, then the much-needed changes across all aspects of our lives can begin and we can start to build a firm foundation with which to leave for future generations to come.

The compiling and penning of this book would not have been possible if I had not have changed the way that I eat, for undoubtedly and without a shadow of a doubt, if I had not have changed my diet, I would be dead.

There is not a day that goes by that I do not give thanks for still being here and living each day as I do.

It becomes abundantly clear and apparent to see how harmful so much food is to us, although with the fast-paced lives that many of us live now, it is all too easy to just grab a snack or a convenience meal, consume it and think no more about it.

Our bodies are our Temples, we are responsible for them and it falls upon us to ensure that how they are run is exemplary. It is up to us to keep them as free and clear from toxins as we possibly can.

None of us would put fuel into our cars if we were unsure of the contents, yet we do this on a daily basis with the most precious vessel we have, which are our bodies, in effect we systematically neglect and abuse the most prized possession we have, yet it is the one we inhabit for life.

I went Vegan after seeing and being part of the vile and archaic system that says we need to consume animals to remain healthy, it took me many years, I got there in the end though.

Having been diagnosed in mid-2015 as having advanced heart failure with multiple life-threatening heart ailments and conditions I became Vegan, which I did solely because of animals. I then began to research into the human health benefits of WFPB, (whole foods plant based) eating.

After many months of intense research, I began to change my diet and eliminated many aspects of foods and additives from it, oils, sugars, fats, processed foods and began to prepare my food from scratch and cook in a different way.

To have faced being told I had no time at all and that in essence I should be dead was horrendous and I would not wish that upon anybody, yet within that heartache, I found a different way, a better and cleaner way to fuel my body.

All of the medication in the world could not have reversed my conditions and sadly, medication is all too often used to merely allow us to cope with an illness rather than addressing the root cause. This is why the pharmaceutical industries and corporations are the biggest money makers in the world, quite simply, there is no money to be made from optimum human health.

I have ravaged my body over the years, pushed it way beyond any and all imaginable limits, yet I am still here and have claimed my health back, not by popping pills, as I am now totally medication free, yet by the realisation that my body is sacred and is my Temple.

I cannot endorse a WFPB way of eating highly enough and I hope that within the words of this book and my experiences, that you will at least think, maybe see and sense the world around you slightly differently and then become more mindful of our place in this Universe.

I dedicate this piece to all of the plant-based Dr's and pioneers of health who are changing the game and paving the way to the realisation that the foods we so readily consume are the best medicines there are and, in my case, and many others, these foods are what have saved our lives and why we are still here today, not just surviving, yet thriving.

Many thanks to all who work tirelessly and are creating the much-needed changes in this world.

These are the Whole Food Plant-based Recipes That Saved My Life

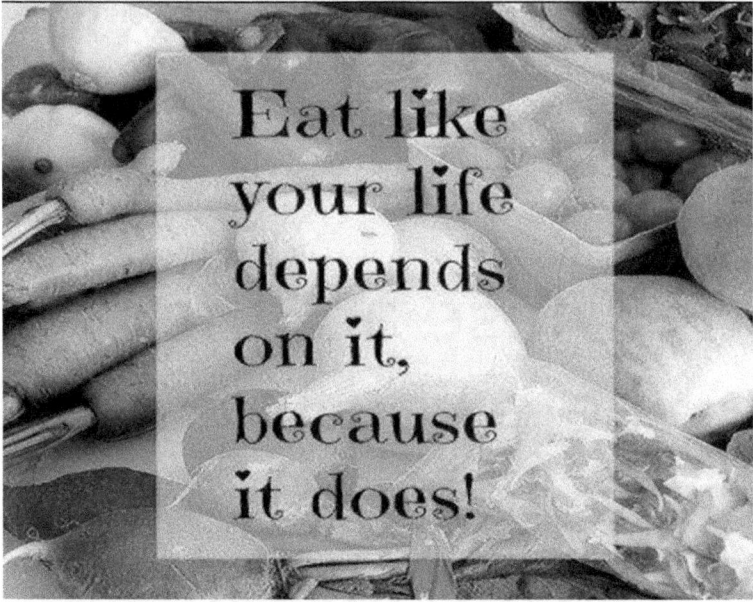

Welcome to the recipe section of this book, all of which are whole foods plant based. Some of these are new recipes which I have devised specifically for this book, whereas others are ones I have been using for ages.,

Here you will find 14 days-worth of breakfasts, lunches and evening meals. All of which are Vegan, (Whole Foods Plant Based) and it is recipes like these that I make and eat the majority of the time.

Not every recipe here is 100% WFPB, there are some ingredients that are minimally processed, yet the majority of these recipes I have created are ranging between 95–99% Whole Foods.

Eating this way has undoubtedly been why and how I have successfully reversed several of the heart ailments, problems and disease which my heart was ravaged with. Having totally transformed the way I live and eat has saved my life and from this, I am now totally medication free and am thriving.

Every recipe provides our bodies with all the goodness and nutrients that we need to survive and live well. All the recipes are perfectly balanced, so please feel free to pick and choose which ones you prefer and as long as you have at least two of these meals a day, then you can rest assured that you will have consumed all that the body needs to power you through each day.

The measurements I use are not specific and are all based on meals for two people, so just increase the amount if you are cooking for larger numbers of people.

I will also include some handy little tips along the way just to pique your interest.

There are no pictures, or elaborate photos that depict the recipes you will be creating, what I want to achieve here is to not give you a comparison to aim for. The meals you create from these recipes will turn out just as they are supposed to, what matters is that you enjoy cooking and experimenting with different flavours and textures.

There are no elaborate ingredients, all these recipes are created from easily obtainable foods and ones which a lot of people will keep as staple foods in their cupboards already.

If I mention an ingredient and you have run out of that, then just replace it with similar. There are no strict stipulations here, just a rough guide which will, hopefully, see you enjoying creating some delicious meals that are all cruelty free, sustainable, vegan and healthy and very tasty.

Breakfasts

Carrot, Apple and Ginger smoothie

Chop up all ingredients into chunks before placing in the blender.

Using a blender or similar, blitz up 1–2 apples, 1–2 carrots and add ginger, depending on taste. Add around 1 pint of Oat, or Soya milk and blitz thoroughly.

This will give you a nice gentle boost and tastes delicious. If you are not versed with creating smoothies, this is a great one to start with as it is so refreshing and packed with nutrients.

* * *

Mashed Avocado on Toast

Carefully remove the stones from 2 Avocados, then using a teaspoon, scrape out the fruit from the outer skin and place into a bowl.

Using a fork to mash, add a pinch of turmeric, pinch of black pepper and mix thoroughly.

Toast two slices of bread slightly, then place the mashed Avocado onto the toast and put under a hot grill until the Avocado starts to brown, then serve.

* * *

Breakfast Buddha Bowl

Prepare a saucepan of porridge using Oat, or Soya milk, then serve into a bowl.

Cover with any fruits you have. I enjoy sliced banana, grated apple, halved strawberries, then a generous sprinkling of Chia seeds and some Cacao powder.

Never be shy in adding more fruit to your breakfast Buddha bowl, as well as creating an array of colour and taste, you are guaranteeing to give yourself a great start to your day.

* * *

Scrambled Tofu

Using a carton of silken smooth Tofu, place the tofu into a dry frying pan and mash with a wooden spoon. Keeping the heat at a medium temperature, add a level teaspoon of Turmeric, a good pinch of black pepper and another level teaspoon of black salt.

Keep stirring and moving around the frying pan, increase heat slightly and keep stirring.

When the tofu is simmering and starting to bubble slightly, then serve. This can be placed onto 2 slices of toast or enjoyed on its own with accompanying fruit, or any left-over veg you may have.

* * *

Fruit with a Side Dip

Fill a bowl with some chopped up, or sliced fruits of your choice.

Drain the aquafaba, (Chickpea water) from a tin, or carton into a blender and add some blueberries, Strawberries or both, then whisk up in the blender until a thick consistency is reached, add more fruit to thicken.

Spoon, or pour over your bowled fruit and enjoy. This puree can also be used to put onto toast and is absolutely delicious.

* * *

Sliced Mushrooms on Toast

Slice several Mushrooms, depending on how many people this is to serve. Place them in a dry saucepan on a low to medium heat, stirring gently. Allow the mushrooms to start sweating, then, whilst stirring, reduce the heat.

These can be served on their own or accompanied with Chickpeas and sprinkled with Nutritional Yeast.

* * *

Overnight Oats

Ideally use a container with a lid, if not available, then use a jug.

Place 1–2 cups of Oats into approx. 1 pint of liquid. This can be either water, a plant milk, or a mixture of both.

Add some quinoa and chia seeds. Shake well or stir and place in a fridge and leave overnight.

In the morning, shake again, or stir, then place into a bowl, add sliced, or finely chopped fruits of your choice if wanted and enjoy a power packed simple breakfast meal.

* * *

Simple Smoothie and toast

Chop up some chunks of watermelon and place into a blender and whisk thoroughly. Add some fresh mint leaves, according to taste, then pour into a highball glass.

Slightly toast 2 slices of bread and the, depending on whether you are a 'lover' or 'hater' spread with Marmite. If you are the latter, then choose another topping for the toast.

I absolutely love this as a breakfast and it's a great start to the day.

* * *

Bubble and Squeak with Scrambled Tofu and Avocado

Mash together any left-over Vegetables you have from a previous meal, place them into a dry frying pan and simmer gently whilst stirring and moving around the pan.

Using the recipe listed for scrambled Tofu, create that in another cook pot and this time, add a mashed-up Avocado to the tofu as well, still adding the turmeric, black pepper and black salt.

This is another quick, yet extremely satisfying and very tasty breakfast.

* * *

Mango and Coconut Water Smoothie

Remove the Mango from the skin and place into a blender, then add Coconut water and blitz thoroughly, then serve into a highball glass and enjoy.

Coconut water is packed with electrolytes and is a superfood. This provides a boost and a great breakfast in a drink.

It is always good to keep a carton of coconut water around. If you feel lethargic, this will help and also if an animal is feeling run down, or showing signs of tiredness, by giving them some coconut water, this will help them and boosts the body as well as the immune system.

* * *

Baked Oatmeal bites

Prepare some overnight Oats whenever you have a spare 5 minutes, making enough for 4 good servings. The consistency needs to be thick, so add more oats to reach the acquired consistency.

Place the oats onto a baking tray lined with foil, the consistency needs to ensure the oats stay together and remain firm.

Bake in an oven on a medium to high heat until nicely brown.

Cut into slices and these are a great standby to keep in the fridge. They can be eaten on their own, or topped with fruits and enjoyed as a breakfast, or as a healthy snack at any time of the day.

* * *

Walnut and Lemon Breakfast Bowl

Using a blender, whisk up a handful of dates, a handful of oats, walnuts, some blueberries, the juice from half a lemon, some chia seeds and cacao powder.

This mixture will be fairly firm, so is ideal to place under the grill to brown off or can be used cold as a base for a breakfast bowl and then topped with sliced banana, apple or strawberries, or whichever fruits you have and prefer.

Whether this is served hot, or cold, sprinkle with some flax, sunflower and pumpkin seeds, then dust with cacao powder and enjoy.

Mashed Chickpea breakfast Punch

Place 1 can, or carton of Chickpeas into a saucepan and add half of the aquafaba, (Chickpea water) into the saucepan.

Allow to simmer slowly and add some whole Cherry, or vine tomatoes. Add 1 teaspoon of Turmeric and a pinch of black pepper and stir gently.

Slowly mash together whilst stirring and allow to break down in the pan.

When cooked, this should be almost paste like and can be served on its own or spread on toast.

Sprinkle with various seeds, Chia, Sunflower, Pumpkin or whatever seeds you have to hand.

* * *

Nut Butter and Fruit Smoothie

Chop up into chunks or pieces an apple, celery and cucumber. Place these into a liquidiser or similar, then add a heaped tablespoon of peanut butter, a few blueberries and a banana.

Add around 1 pint of plant milk and blitz thoroughly until a fairly thick consistency is reached.

Serve into a highball glass to drink on its own or use as a nice topping for any Baked Oatmeal Bites you may have to hand.

* * *

FACT

Oat milk is ranked Number 1 on all sustainability metrics.

Lunches and Light Bites

Sweet Potato, Green Pepper and Leek Soup

Chop the ingredients into fairly small pieces and place into a saucepan and almost cover with water.

Add a teaspoon of turmeric and a good pinch of black pepper. Put in a generous sprinkling of dried mixed herbs and allow to slowly simmer on a medium heat whilst stirring occasionally.

As the potato starts to break down, use a potato masher to mix up and mash all together whilst still remaining on the heat.

Continue to stir and if this reduces too quickly, then add some plant milk of your choice.

Use the potato masher again until you reach the required texture, chunky or not so, the choice is yours.

Allow this to simmer further whilst stirring and then serve when ready.

Baked Potato and Beans

Oven bake a couple of potatoes, normal spuds, or sweet potatoes. Slicing them halfway through lengthways and sideways, effectively cutting an X into them from top to bottom as this allows them to cook more evenly.

Empty a can of baked beans into a saucepan once the potatoes are almost ready. I always add a splash of Oat milk to my baked beans as this gives a slightly creamier texture. Add a spoonful of Marmite, if required, to the beans and add a teaspoon of turmeric and a pinch of black pepper also.

Place the beans on a medium heat and stir.

Once the potatoes are ready, remove from the oven and were they have been cut, prise them open and place on a plate.

Drizzle the baked beans over the potatoes or add as a side accompaniment. Sprinkle with Chia seeds, nutritional yeast and enjoy.

* * *

Stuffed Peppers (Capsicums)

Place 1 can, or carton of chickpeas including the aquafaba into a saucepan and add a handful of quinoa to it also and place onto a medium heat.

Carefully cut around the stalk of 1 or 2 Peppers, remove and then use a teaspoon to scrape out the seeds and pith from inside.

Whilst the Chickpea mixture is simmering nicely and reducing in liquid, dice up 2 mushrooms and place into the saucepan along with a few halved tomatoes. Add turmeric, black pepper and mixed herbs and stir.

Once the liquid is reduced and the tomatoes have broken down, spoon the mixture into the Peppers and if you kept the stalk, place it back on top.

Put both Peppers in a medium heat oven and allow to slowly cook further.

When done, carefully remove from the oven, place on a plate and serve with a small mixed salad of your choice.

* * *

Buddha Bowl Salad

Tear up some lettuce leaves, dice some onions, then mix together using a fork, or your hands, then place this into a serving dish, or bowl.

Slice some beetroot, grate a couple of carrots, thinly slice a few tomatoes and cucumber, then place these on top of the lettuce and onion mixture.

Drizzle with the juice of half a lemon or lime, then sprinkle with various seeds, nutritional yeast and serve with sliced bread or toast.

* * *

Quinoa Warm and Cold Salad

Simmer around 4 cups of quinoa in a saucepan and allow to bubble gently.

In another saucepan, blanche some Kale and courgettes. Don't allow these to get anywhere near boiling point as the firmness needs to be kept.

Once the quinoa is ready, it doesn't take long at all, drain off all the residual water then place back on the cooker hob with the heat turned off. The slight heat just gets rid of any water that is left, so stir constantly.

Add the kale and sliced courgettes into the saucepan with the quinoa in, stir again and add the juice from half a lime, or lemon, then stir again then serve into a bowl.

Sprinkle on some cashew nuts and some Chia seeds, then add some satsuma/tangerine segments, mix together and enjoy a taste sensation.

* * *

> **FACT**
>
> Turmeric is a superfood and a great antioxidant for our bodies. The active and powerful ingredient in Turmeric is called Curcumin and this is known to help alleviate arthritis, cure cancers and has many other health benefits also.
>
> Our bodies struggle to absorb Turmeric fully, yet a sure-fire way to gain all that we can from this super-food, is to add black pepper with it each time you use it.
>
> The piperine, the active ingredient in black pepper, reacts with the curcumin and our bodies can then absorb it by up to 2,000% more efficiently.

Bean and Salad Pittas

Place half a carton of kidney beans along with a small handful of red and green lentils into a saucepan, using the liquid from the kidney beans as a stock.

Dice about 2 good sized mushrooms and place into the same saucepan and then set to a medium heat.

Cut about 5–6 small tomatoes in half, then put those into the saucepan also and stir gently allowing the ingredients to move around whilst heating and reducing the stock.

Chop a small onion into pieces, shred some lettuce leaves and dice a small piece of cucumber. Place all of these into a bowl and then mix these by hand, or fork and leave on the side.

Use wholewheat Pitta bread and gently prise them open, 2–3 pittas will be needed here.

Once the stock in the saucepan is almost all gone, drain off any that is left, then mix the bean and lentil mix in with the salad and stir together.

Using a dessert spoon, load the bean, lentil and salad mix into the pittas and enjoy a nutritionally packed lunch.

* * *

Baked Veg and Oil Free Chips

Cut 2 large potatoes, normal, sweet, or both into chunky chip size pieces, then place on a rack on a baking tray.

Sprinkle lightly with crushed garlic and black pepper then place in a pre-heated oven set to 180C high temperature.

Being on a rack means the chips will bake evenly and come out crispy on the outside and fluffy on the inside, this will take between 30–45 mins depending on temperature and oven.

Slice into lengths, a couple of carrots, parsnips, peppers, any veg you have to hand and after the chips have been cooking for around 15 minutes, then place all the other veg onto the baking tray and around the rack which the chips are on.

Test a chip after between 30–45 mins and if it's done, then serve all the veg and chips together on a plate or in a bowl and enjoy a taste explosion.

* * *

Cauliflower, Lentil and Onion Soup with Tofu Croutons

Chop up one small cauliflower into florets and slice the inner stalk into chunks, then place these into a good-sized saucepan.

Add a handful of lentils, red or green, whichever you have or prefer, into the same pan and then chop 1 medium sized onion and place that into the saucepan also, then almost cover with water and place onto a medium heat and allow to start simmering.

Using a block of firm Tofu, chop this into dice sized pieces, then place on a baking tray and put into a medium heat oven, turning occasionally until all are golden brown and crisp to the touch, then remove from oven and leave on the side.

Using a potato masher, mash up the cauliflower, lentil and onion soup to a preferred consistency. Keep simmering to reduce the liquid content and if need be, turn the temperature up whilst stirring constantly.

When the soup has reduced enough, serve into a bowl, sprinkle with turmeric, black pepper, add some of the baked tofu croutons and then enjoy some hearty, wholesome and delicious soup.

* * *

Mushroom and Onion Scramble with Cauliflower Wings

Use a good size Cauliflower and slice into thick wedges cutting from the head down to the stalk, then slice again into half pieces.

Brush, or dip into a plant-based milk and then dust with turmeric, black pepper, chilli flakes and breadcrumbs, then place on a baking tray in a medium temperature oven for around 30–40 minutes.

Dice up 1 medium sized onion and about 4 good sized mushrooms.

Using 1 carton, 200g, of silken smooth Tofu, cook in a dry pan and add the mushrooms and onion and keep moving around the pan until cooked.

Remove the Cauliflower Wings from the oven, place on a plate and serve with the mushroom and onion scramble and top off with breadcrumbs if you have some left over, then simply eat and enjoy.

* * *

Pasta with Home-made Sauce

Place a good serving of whole wheat pasta into a saucepan of well simmering water, stir occasionally and don't allow to boil.

Chop 6 large tomatoes in half, slice 2 celery sticks into small pieces and cut 2 apples into chunks. Place these into a blender and mix thoroughly. Add the juice of 1 lime into this, along with some black pepper and mix again.

When the pasta is ready, drain off all the water, serve into a bowl and drizzle with the home-made sauce.

Pasta is always a good stand by to have in your cupboards, as well as being high in carbohydrates, eating pasta is like a happy drug as it raises our serotonin levels and makes us feel more positive and vibrant.

* * *

Creamy Mash

Potatoes are so versatile and there is something extremely comforting about a nice serving of mashed potatoes.

Chop up 3 large normal potatoes and 3 large, sweet potatoes, keep the skins on as they contain so much goodness.

Allow to simmer gently on a medium heat for around 18–20 minutes, or when they appear to be starting to fall apart. Drain all the water off and then add 1 cup of Oat, or Soya milk, some black pepper, diced onions, diced mushrooms and some chopped chives.

Mash together thoroughly and obtain the consistency you require, lumpy, or smooth, it's up to you.

This creamy mash is a meal in itself or can be used as part of a larger meal.

* * *

Chickpea and Courgette Soup

Using a carton or can of Chickpeas (feel free to pre-soak dried ones if you prefer, I do both and cartons/cans are convenient) place the contents, including all the aquafaba into a saucepan and place on a medium heat.

Add some paprika, according to taste, a pinch of black pepper and stir.

Slice 1–2 Courgettes and place those into the saucepan also.

Allow to simmer gradually and, using a potato masher, mash up the chickpeas and courgettes. You may have to repeat this 2–3 times until it is a thick consistency, allowing the liquid to reduce enough.

When the soup is ready, serve into a bowl, sprinkle with any seeds that you have and serve with whole meal, or seeded bread, or toast.

* * *

FACT

When we consume Iron rich foods, tofu, chickpeas, lentils, kale, seeds and many others, our bodies can struggle to absorb the Iron contained within them. To help this and increase our bodies absorption rate, it is always good to eat some Vitamin C afterwards. This can be obtained from a variety of sources, including, oranges, kiwi fruit, Bell peppers, spinach and Brussel sprouts to name a few.

Crispy Banana toast with Salad

This is so easy to make and is great as a lunch meal, or a quick snack.

Take 2 good sized bananas which are starting to blacken on the outside skin, these are sweeter to taste and creamier to eat.

Mash them up in a bowl using a fork, add a pinch of cinnamon and mix thoroughly.

Slightly toast 2 slices of seeded whole meal bread and then, using a knife, spread the banana mix onto the toast, then place under a medium heat grill for around 3–5 minutes.

Slice up some raw carrots, mushrooms, a pepper and some cucumber, then sprinkle with some Chia and other seeds and use this as a side dish for the banana toast.

After 3–5 minutes, remove the banana toast from the grill and enjoy another tasty and nutritionally rich meal.

Spinach, Quinoa and Red Pepper Salad

Place 2 handfuls of washed Quinoa into a saucepan, then cover with water and allow to simmer on a medium heat, stirring frequently for 15 mins.

Crumble 1 Kalo low salt stock cube into the saucepan, along with a pinch of turmeric, black pepper and a few chilli flakes, still allowing it to simmer and reduce.

Lay a nice bed of fresh spinach leaves into a bowl, then once ready and drained, place the quinoa on top of the spinach leaves.

Slice into strips one red pepper and place that on top, or alongside the quinoa, then serve and enjoy.

* * *

Evening Meals, (Dinner)

Rainbow Stir Fry Veg with Noodles

Using a wok, or a deep-frying pan, both of which need a lid to cover them, place on a medium heat and add a minimal amount of Soya, or Oat milk, just to thinly cover the bottom of the pan.

Throw in whichever veg you have to hand, whether that is fresh, or frozen, (sadly frozen veg are often fresher than unfrozen veg as the flavour is locked in within hours of being picked and airmiles are often avoided to some degree.)

Make the stir fry a rainbow of colour and as we eat with our eyes first, this is essential. Try to use an array of veg, carrots, peas, sweetcorn, courgettes, mushrooms, broccoli, peppers are always good as well, (peppers are a fruit) as they give a different texture and are so vibrant in colour.

Place some lentils, quinoa, or bulgur wheat into the pan also, these add another dimension entirely and are so good for us.

If you have some raisins, or sultanas close by, place some into the stir fry also.

Add 1 Kalo low salt vegetable stock cube to the pan, a pinch of black pepper, some turmeric and some chilli flakes.

Keep stirring at regular intervals and after about 15 mins of cooking, place some free from dairy and egg noodles into the pan and cover for 5 minutes with the lid.

Remove the lid and the noodles should start to stir in with the vegetables nicely now. Stir every minute or so and then cover in between stirring.

By ow, the noodles should be heated through enough, some of the veg will be turning slightly golden brown and will still have a nice crunch to them.

Remove from the heat and serve into bowls, or dishes. Feel free to sprinkle breadcrumbs and/or seeds and then enjoy.

* * *

Slo – Cooker Winter Warmer Hot Pot

A slo – cooker is great if you have one and you can use these for an array of dishes.

For this I use TVP (textured vegetable protein) a Vegan/plant based dried mince alternative. Place 2–3 cups into the pot, add some dry vegetable gravy powder to this, mixed herbs, a bay leaf or 2, black pepper and some turmeric.

Fill the slo – cooker up to about two thirds full of an assortment of Vegetables, (fresh or frozen,) sliced mushrooms, peas, carrots, broccoli and cauliflower florets, green beans, sweetcorn and sliced courgettes.

This now needs to be about half filled with liquid, the TVP dried mince soaks a lot of moisture up as do the gravy granules.

I use a mixture of Oat milk and hot water, then add until the cooking pot is around half filled.

Stir thoroughly and if you are leaving this all day, turn onto a medium heat. If you are at home, or coming back, stir again if possible.

After around 8 hours of cooking gradually, the aroma from this will fill your house and give you a fantastic evening meal to come home too.

When ready, turn off the power, serve on its own, or sprinkle with Tofu croutons and then enjoy.

* * *

Vegetable Curry with Rice

Place whatever Vegetables you have, or fancy, into a deep saucepan, along with a block of silken smooth Tofu.
Add herbs and curry powder according to taste.

Add some hot water and plant milk, best to do this gradually and place pan on a medium heat.

Allow to simmer slowly for 2–3 hours and stir occasionally.

As the curry begins to form and the liquid reduces, add some dates, dried apricots and some goji berries, stir again and reduce the heat slightly until a very gentle simmer is happening.

Brown rice is my personally choice, although feel free to use your preferred rice.

Put a saucepan of water on to boil and whilst waiting for that, place the rice in a large sieve and gently run it under the tap, this gets rid of a lot of the starch from the rice.

When the pan of water is just about boiling, place the rice into it and leave for about 45 mins, 18 mins for white rice and 12 mins for basmati.

Once the rice is cooked, serve onto a plate, either as a bed for the curry, or on one side, serve the curry and then top with chopped walnuts, and/or brazil nuts, accompany with a garnish of spinach leaves and then enjoy a texture and taste explosion.

* * *

Oil Free Falafels with Salad

Drain 1 tin/carton of Chickpeas and place them into a
blender, add 1 cup of Chickpea flour, 1 diced onion, 1 level
teaspoon of turmeric, a good pinch of black pepper,
1 medium sized onion which has been diced, then add
2 cloves of garlic which have been crushed.

Blend this all together, then add 1 handful of Oats, the juice
from half a lime, 3 tablespoons of tahini paste and some fresh
herbs to taste.

Once blended together, scrape out onto a plate, this should
be like a firm dough mixture now, (if the mixture is too dry,
just add a little warm water.) Mould into round balls, bite sized
and place onto a foil lined baking tray.

Preheat the oven to a high temperature and place them into
the oven. Turn them over after about 20 minutes, then place
back into the oven and leave for another 20 minutes.

Serve with a sliced salad of carrots strips, torn lettuce,
radishes which have been halved, sliced tomatoes and then
drizzle the salad and falafels with the juice of the other half of
the lime.

* * *

Roasted Asparagus with Roast Potatoes Oil Free Recipe

Chop 4 large potatoes, normal, sweet or both into large chunks and place onto a rack which is seated on a baking tray. These are going to be dry roasted the same way as the chips from an earlier recipe were cooked.

Once on the rack, place them into a hot oven and then leave for 30 mins.

After 30 minutes, remove the baking tray with the rack on it and place the Asparagus spears onto the baking tray and around the rack. Dust with garlic powder, turmeric and black pepper, then return all to the oven.

Allow all this to cook for approx. 15 minutes and then remove from oven. The Potatoes should now be crispy on the outside and fluffy in the centre and the asparagus should be just starting to brown slightly.

Serve onto a plate, drizzle the asparagus spears with lime, or lemon juice, then sprinkle with chia and sunflower seeds and enjoy a tasty, crispy and oil free meal.

* * *

Chunky Bite Buddha Bowl

Cook a good serving of rice, around 4 handfuls, or enough for 2 servings.

Chop into dice sized chunks, 2 medium sized sweet potatoes and one carton of firm Tofu.

Place these into a medium heat oven and then turn every 10 minutes until golden brown and ready.

Slice 1 red and 1 green pepper into strips. Chop 3 carrots and one apple into chunks.

When the rice is cooked, serve into 2 bowls as the Buddha bowl bed. Take the sweet potato and tofu chunks and place on top of the rice, then lay the sliced peppers, carrots and apple chunks on also.

Scatter with raisins, sultanas and seeds you have to hand, then eat and enjoy.

* * *

Butternut Squash, Kale and Carrot Soup with Noodles

Carefully remove the skin from the butternut squash, I find an old-fashioned potato peeler works well for this. Once peeled, cut into chunks and place in a large saucepan.

Chop up about 6 medium sized carrots, place those into the pan and then add 4 good handfuls of kale.

Almost cover with water, place on a medium heat and allow to reduce slowly.

Add turmeric, black pepper and stir gently.

After this has been simmering for around 30 minutes, mash up with a potato masher and continue heating and mashing until this has nicely reduced to a thick soup consistency.

Leave on a low to medium heat and add some dairy and egg free noodles, we are aiming for 2 servings here, so add the amount you feel is right for 2 people.

Stir gently for around 15–20 minutes, or until the noodles are cooked, raising the heat if needed.

Once cooked, serve into 2 bowls and sprinkle with chia seeds, a pinch of black pepper, some spinach leaves and accompany with seeded bread, or toast.

* * *

Layered Shepherdless Pie

Using a large saucepan or pot, add 2–3 cups of TVP mince, 1 can, or carton of chopped tomatoes, 6 sliced mushrooms, 2 chopped celery stalks, 2 handfuls of red/green lentils, 1 sliced yellow pepper and 3 chopped carrots.

Add about half a pint of plant milk, (Oat or Soya) and then add the same amount of water to the mixture stir thoroughly.

Crumble up 2 Kalo low salt Vegetable stock cubes and add those. Add 1 teaspoon of turmeric, 2 pinches of black pepper,

1 bay leaf and a good sprinkling of mixed herbs. Stir again and place on a medium heat. Whilst cooking, if the mix appears, or seems dry, add more plant milk and water accordingly and allow to slowly simmer.

This mixture can be left on a medium heat for between 2–3 hours with occasional stirring.

Slice up 3–4 courgettes and allow to simmer in a saucepan of water for around 5 minutes ensuring they retain a slight crunch, then remove from the water, place onto a plate and leave on the side.

Chop up 3 medium sized potatoes and 3 medium sized sweet potatoes, place these into a saucepan, cover with water and heat on a medium heat and allow to simmer for about 20 minutes, or until slightly soft.

Once ready, drain the water from the potatoes, add a good splash of plant milk a pinch of black pepper and mash until a nice creamy texture is reached.

The large TVP mix should be ready now, so place some of it into a glass, or similar dish to go into the oven.

Layer this with the courgettes from earlier, then add more of the TVP mixture on top. Spoon, or fork the mashed potatoes on the very top, sprinkle evenly with black pepper, then place into a hot oven and leave for between 35–45 minutes depending on oven type and temperature.

Once ready, serve into bowls, or plates and enjoy this delicious cruelty free Layered Shepherdless Pie.

Baked Jackfruit and Pasta

Using a can, (fresh if you have it) drain the water and fork out the Jackfruit from the can into a medium sized saucepan and add about 100ml of Oat, or Soya milk and place onto a medium heat.

Add around 1 cup of sweetcorn, some sliced green beans and 6–8 cherries, or vine tomatoes along with some chilli flakes and a pinch of garlic salt.

In another saucepan, put in enough wholewheat pasta, enough for 2 people to have a good serving each, then cover with water and place on a medium – high heat and allow to simmer for around 2 minutes.

Using 1 cup of plant milk and some chickpea flour, mix up and whisk thoroughly until you have a fairly thick mixture that is pourable.

Dice up 1 small onion and 4 large mushrooms, then place this into the plant milk and flour mix and leave on the side.

Once the pasta is cooked, drain off the water, then empty into the pan that contains the Jackfruit and other ingredients. Turn the heat up slightly and stir it all together until the liquid has reduced significantly.

Using a large baking tray, empty the Jackfruit, Pasta and veg into the tray and spread out evenly, then pour the flour and plant milk mix over the pasta, place into the oven and allow to bake for around 20–30 minutes.

Once the pasta starts to go a golden-brown colour, the dish is ready to serve.

Add some fresh salad on the plate as an accompaniment and enjoy.

* * *

Fruit Bowl with Drizzle

Take a mango, 2 bananas, some dates, (with stones removed) 2 small oranges, 2 apples, 2 pears, a handful of strawberries and some assorted nuts.

Peel, chop and slice the various fruits, and nuts, then evenly place into 2 separate bowls.

Take around 100 ml of plant milk, place into a jug, or mixing bowl and then place a small punnet/tray of blueberries and either mix with a fork, or use a handhold blitzer and whisk thoroughly, this is now the drizzle for the bowled fruit, and this makes a delicious meal in itself.

Feel free to sprinkle any seeds and extra nuts on the top if you fancy, then enjoy a totally delicious and very vibrant fruit bowl.

* * *

Power Packed Wholewheat Wraps

Slowly simmer 3 handfuls of quinoa and 2 handfuls of green lentils in a saucepan, keep stirring and allow this to cook for between 20–30 minutes, depending on heat, then when ready, drain off all the water and empty into a large sieve, shaking this will get rid of any extra liquid, then empty into a bowl.

Slice 2 good sized carrots, half a cucumber and half of a courgette into long thin strips, (julienne) then place these into a bowl, sprinkle with ginger, black pepper and chilli flakes, then mix all these around slightly.

Take 4 wholewheat wraps and lay onto a worksurface. Carefully lay the sliced veg along the middle, ensuring you will be able to fold and wrap them sufficiently.

Mix up the green lentil and quinoa mixture and lay this on top of the sliced veg, then carefully fold the wraps and then cut them in half to be left with 8 separate and tasty Power Packed Wholewheat wraps.

Accompany with a side salad if required, then enjoy this crunchy and tasty treat.

* * *

HANDY TIP

There are normally 2 reasons why we get headaches. 1 of those can be that our bodies are dehydrated, which is easily done, and the truth is, once we feel thirsty, we are already dehydrating.

The other reason we suffer headaches is that we are lacking vital minerals and a good thing here is to take a pinch of either rock, or sea salt and place directly under the tongue and allow to dissolve on its own.

Tofu and Vegetable Pan Bake

A solid cast-iron deep-frying pan is good for this, as ideally, the pan needs to be placed into the oven to finish. If you haven't got one suitable, then use an ordinary pan to start with and just prepare a baking tray for the end part.

Chop 1 block of firm tofu into chunks, along with 2 sweet potatoes, 1 courgette, 3 carrots, 1 small broccoli head and place into a dry frying pan on a medium heat.

Add 1 clove of crushed garlic, a pinch of paprika, black pepper and a generous sprinkle of mixed herbs.

Add 100ml of plant milk to the pan and keep stirring and allow the plant milk to gently simmer and keep this on the heat for 20–30 minutes.

If you are using the same pan to place into the oven, carefully tip the pan to one side and spoon the liquid over the tofu and veg to keep it moist on the top.

If you are unable to use the same pan, then transfer the tofu and veg onto a baking tray, then pour the liquid over the top that way.

Place into a high temperature oven for 20–30 minutes, then remove from the oven, serve onto 2 plates, or bowls, garnish with a side salad if desired, then sprinkle with various seeds, some breadcrumbs and enjoy.

* * *

Baked Chestnut Mushrooms and Walnuts

You will need 8 large Chestnut mushrooms for this, along with 2 handfuls of walnuts, some salad leaves and some grated coconut.

Place the 8 Chestnut mushrooms onto 1, or 2 baking trays and place in the oven on a medium temperature for around 30 minutes.

Depending on the temperature and efficiency of your oven, you might need to rotate the baking trays once or twice during the cooking process.

Once the mushrooms are baked nicely, remove from the oven, then place the walnuts onto the baking tray/trays, then sprinkle the mushrooms with the grated coconut.

There should be some liquid in the trays from the mushrooms, carefully spoon this over the mushrooms and return to the oven for a further 10 minutes.

Remove from the oven, serve onto 2 plates/bowls in equal amounts and then garnish with a side salad and bon Appetit.

* * *

Buddha Power Bowl

Oven bake 3 large, sweet potatoes and when cooked, cut into chunks and leave in the side to cool down.

Lay a thick bed of mixed salad leaves into 2 bowls, then on top of the leaves, place, sliced beetroot, sliced red and green peppers, 2 avocado halves, some chopped tomatoes, carrot strips and then scatter the baked sweet potato chunks over each bowl.

Add whichever seeds you fancy, or have to hand and serve with either toasted, seeded bread, or untoasted bread.

This is a protein and nutrient dense Buddha bowl of goodness which will give you a power boost, so enjoy.

* * *

I have certainly enjoyed writing this book and I hope that you have enjoyed the journey, regardless of how hard it may have been to read at times?

I have poured my very being into these pages and they contain my very heart, soul and essence, all here to be read, absorbed, learnt from and hopefully you will be comforted and inspired.

Thank you for reading my words and feeling my inner being and scars.

This life is so very precious, all that we have is this moment in time, anything past this point is a rich blessing and not guaranteed.

As we all venture onwards, we need to cherish each moment, savour every second and walk valiantly onwards without trepidation, for we have this one life and this is it, there is no practice run.

Each one of us has great potential and drive within us and it falls upon us as individuals to be the changes that we wish to see in this world and in leading by example, we can help to create a better world, not just for ourselves, but for all beings and all species.

For we are the Guardians and Caretakers of this world and we know better, so now is the time that we start to be and do better, for if not us, who else is there?

I wish you all much love and peace and I hope my words have touched you in some way, maybe made you think, who knows, I certainly hope so.

Please feel free to contact me and you will find my contact details on my website: **johnawen.com**

Thank you.

John Awen

CENTRE OF EXCELLENCE
AWARDS
— 2020 —
HIGHLY COMMENDED

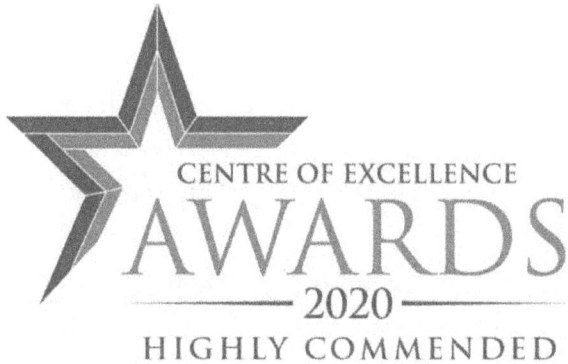

John Awen has faced many trials in his life, yet with sheer resilience and dogged determination he has risen up to not only face his challenges, but has fought to overcome them. Having overcome a huge drug addiction, reversed life-threatening heart disease, he then turned his life around to become a multiple published author, nutritionist and public speaker. Having been nominated for an award in the Inspiration category for the prestigious Centre of Excellence Awards in 2020, he became a finalist and went on to win the coveted Highly Commended accolade in the Inspiration category.

John Awen's short and pungent story, like the return journey of Odysseus to Ithaca, is a tortured experience.

John's "Troy" was the hell of his own creation; a life-threatening addiction to drugs; theft and other avenues of law-breaking; and several close encounters with death.

But in the end, his "Odyssey" is enlightened and redemptive.

I was struck by John's brutal honesty. He holds himself personally and exclusively responsible for his actions and their consequences, seeking neither sympathy and forgiveness.

His book is simplicity itself; laying out the cards, describing how he played them, and lost; and how he chose to stop playing.

One phrase in his short story stood out for me.

"Fear and Guilt"

John asserts, without needing to explain, that these are self-destructive forces.

Reading his words reminded me of my boyhood, reading Alexandre Dumas' masterpiece, "The Count of Monte Cristo".

"All human wisdom is contained in two words, "Wait and Hope".

John discovers, through his own visceral experiences, the carnage inflicted on innocent, powerless animals.

He employs two new verbs, without stating them explicitly.

"Decide" and "Act".

He "Decides" to reject cruelty, becoming Vegan;

He "Acts" to become an Animal Rights Advocate.

His metamorphosis is stunning.

The changes in the man are not simply reflected in his diet, lifestyle or beliefs.

Rather, they describe his "Character", and a civilized mind.

The effects on his life are palpable.

The consequences for the powerless are immeasurable.

Philip Wollen

Lightning Source UK Ltd.
Milton Keynes UK
UKHW020420200221
379018UK00006B/202

9 781916 014091